DATE DUE

JUN 01 '98

C
Is
for   *ry*

HIGHSMITH # 45220

Gerontological Nursing: Issues and Opportunities for the Twenty-First Century

Mary Burke and Susan Sherman, Editors

National League for Nursing Press • New York
Pub. No. 14-2510

Copyright © 1993
National League for Nursing Press
350 Hudson Street, New York, NY 10014

All rights reserved. No part of this book may be reproduced in print, or by photostatic means, or in any other manner, without the express written permission of the publisher.

ISBN 0-88737-572-3

> The views expressed in this publication represent the views of the authors and do not necessarily reflect the official views of the National League for Nursing Press.

Library of Congress Cataloging-in-Publication Data

Gerontological nursing : issues and opportunities for the twenty-first century / Mary Burke and Susan Sherman, editors.
    p.   cm.
  Includes bibliographical references.
  Pub. no. 14-2510
  ISBN 0-88737-572-3
  1. Geriatric nursing. 2. Nursing home care. 3. Nursing education. I. Burke, Mary M. II. Sherman, Susan, RN.
  [DNLM: 1. Geriatric Nursing—trends—congresses. WY 152 G3772]
RC954.G478 1993
610.73'65—dc20
DNLM/DLC
for Libary of Congress   92-48261
                                                                CIP

This book was set in Goudy by Publications Development Company of Texas. The editor and designer was Allan Graubard. The cover was designed by Lauren Stevens. Northeastern Press was the printer and binder.

Printed in the United States of America

Contents

	Contributors	vii
	Preface	ix
	Forward	xi
	Introduction	xiii
1.	Gerontological Nursing Issues and Opportunities for Twenty-First Century "Not for the Weak of Heart: The Politics of Long-Term Care" *Sister Rosemary Donley*	1
2.	Issues and Opportunities for the Twenty-First Century: The Search for a Definition of Quality in Long Term Care Settings *Donna A. Peters*	13
3.	New Practice Models in Long-Term Care *Christine Heine and Sister Rose Therese Bahr*	27
4.	The Nursing Home Clinical: New Horizons for Capitalizing on a Caring Experience *M. Elaine Tagliareni*	37
5.	Relationships in Clinical Teaching: The Faculty Role Revisited *Verle Waters*	45
6.	Gerontologic Nursing Competency Development: Associate Degree in Nursing & Bachelor of Science in Nursing: History—Commonalities—Differences *Susan Sherman and Mary Burke*	51
7.	Facilitating Student Learning: Effective Teaching Strategies for Baccalaureate Education *Norma R. Small*	61

8.	About Anger and Power	69
	Patricia Moccia	
9.	A Symphony of Caring: Shared Visions and Eloquent Futures for Nursing Education and Practice	81
	Em Olivia Bevis	

Contributors

Sister Rose Therese Bahr, ASC, PhD, RN, FAAN, is Former Professor of Nursing, School of Nursing, The Catholic University of America, Washington, DC.

Em Olivia Bevis, EdD, RN, FAAN, is Consultant in Nursing Education and Adjunct Professor, Research, Georgia Southern University, Statesboro, Georgia.

Mary Burke, DNSc, RN, CANP, is Director, Gerontologic Nursing Program, School of Nursing, Georgetown University, Washington, DC.

Sister Rosemary Donley, PhD, RN, FAAN, is Executive Vice President, The Catholic University of America, Washington, DC.

Christine Heine, MS, RN, C, is Visiting Assistant Professor, School of Nursing, University of North Carolina-Chapel Hill.

Patricia Moccia, PhD, RN, FAAN, is Chief Operating Officer, National League for Nursing, New York, New York.

Donna A. Peters, PhD, RN, FAAN, is Project Director, In Search of Excellence in Home Care Project, Community Health Accreditation Program, New York, New York.

Susan Sherman, MA, RN, is Head, Department of Nursing, Community College of Philadelphia, Philadelphia, Pennsylvania, National Project Administrator, Community College–Nursing Home Partnership.

Norma R. Small, PhD, CRNP, is Coordinator for Sponsored Projects, School of Nursing, Georgetown University, Washington, DC.

Elaine M. Tagliareni, is Associate Professor, Community College of Philadelphia, Philadelphia, Pennsylvania.

Verle Waters, is Dean Emerita, Ohlone College, Freemont, California, and Project Consultant, Community College–Nursing Home Partnership.

Preface

The 1992 conference, Gerontological Nursing: Issues and Opportunities for the Twenty-First Century, held in San Diego and Chicago, was an outcome of the collaborative effort of faculty from the Community College–Nursing Home Partnership Dissemination Project, funded by the W.K. Kellogg Foundation, Georgetown University Gerontologic Nursing Graduate program, and the National League for Nursing. The goal of the conference was to bring together nursing faculty from community college and university programs with clinicians from acute and long-term care. The three objectives of the conference were: to foster a sense of collegiality, to share ideas, and to establish a vision for the future.

In the less than perfect world of health care, the nation's frail elderly, particularly those who reside in nursing homes, are at risk for diminished services. There exists unprecedented opportunities for nursing to improve the quality of health care services received by this growing population. This challenge can be seen as the moral imperative that joins nurses in a common struggle.

The papers are organized to discuss gerontolgic nursing within educational, clinical, and political perspectives. Included in the proceedings are papers of interest to a wide audience of nursing educators and clinicians.

The editors wish to acknowledge Dr. Helen Grace from the W.K. Kellogg Foundation for her vision and unwavering support for Community College–Nursing Home Projects, Verle Waters for her elegant ability to care, Sister Rose Theresa Bahr for her gentle prodding of the collaborative effort between faculty from Georgetown University and from the Community College–Nursing Home Partnership, Dr. Patricia Moccia, Chief Operating Officer, National League for Nursing, for her commitment to gerontologic nursing, and last but not least to Sally Barhydt, Managing Editor and Assistant Vice President for Communications, National League for Nursing, for her extraordinary talents in bringing this book to completion.

Mary Burke DNSc, RN, CANP
Susan Sherman MA, RN

Forward

Preparation of nurses to serve older adults in the United States requires a curricular design based on scientific knowledge and skills/competencies that provide a firm foundation for the complexities of care needed by this population. When this foundation is begun in the associate degree nursing program, extended into the baccalaureate degree program, and advanced in graduate programs in the speciality of gerontological nursing the recipients of care, the older adults, are the beneficiaries. With the growing numbers of older persons who will need nursing care in future years it is critical that nurse educators, from academic settings who are charged with the preparation of gerontological nurses at all levels, and nurse practitioners, from the service sector who are the providers of care in institutional and community-based settings, analyze the care needs of older adults in contemporary society. With the data from each of these important players a curricular design based on experiential as well as scientific data emerges. It is with pleasure that I acknowledge the collaborative efforts of Georgetown University School of Nursing faculty and the project directors and faculty of the Community College of Pennsylvania for implementing a suggestion advanced at one of the Advisory Board meetings regarding a joint venture for better preparation of gerontological nurses. This joint venture occurred in San Diego, California, and Chicago, Illinois, when the National League for Nursing sponsored joint meetings of these two educational institutions and nurses engaged in preparation of gerontological nurses. The conferences were well attended and highly praised for initiating a pioneering work in gerontological nursing.

This publication demonstrates the efforts of these two educational institutions to promote a collaborative relationship for preparation of gerontological nurses. The content of the conference provides important information on curricular issues and designs with far-reaching effects in the future. I am grateful to the faculty of the two institutions who provided me with the opportunity to be involved in this important and historic event. On behalf of the millions of older adults who will be influenced by excellent nursing care as a result of this joint effort, I offer my best wishes to all conference presenters and present readers. Because of this joint effort, the cause of the gerontological nursing has been advanced significantly. As a result, this publication is a must for nursing school libraries, nurse practitioner bookshelves, deans of schools of nursing and their faculties, and administrators of long-term care health facilities and community health agencies.

Sister Rose Therese Bahr, ASC, PhD, RN, FAAN
Former Professor of Nursing
The Catholic University of America
School of Nursing
Washington, DC

Introduction:
Convening the Conference: Day 1

Verle Waters

In convening this conference, it seemed unlikely that I would speak of demographics. The present audience is a select group, already interested in the topic, and have heard and read many times over the numbers which justify our interest in gerontologic issues and opportunities for the twenty-first century. Recently, however, I read some figures that surprised me as they might you. In America, 29 million people are older than 65; in Russia, 26 million people live past this benchmark; in India and on the Asian continent 33 million people are over 65; and in China, 53 million people are over 65.

Facts such as these are no longer merely interesting. We live on a shrinking planet, and our fortunes are increasingly linked to world affairs. Our educational programs graduate men and women who will practice nursing for 30, 40, or more years in the twenty-first century, serving a society that has new borders, or no borders. Not long ago, I took a telephone call from a nursing faculty member at the University of Tel Aviv who learned, while in the United States, about the Community College–Nursing Home project. She was seeking information about the teaching of gerontology in the nursing curriculum because of rapid change in the population of Israel. One-fourth of the massive migration of immigrants to Israel from the Soviet Union is over 65, flooding health services with a geriatric population that has suffered years of health care neglect. And the nursing school curriculum is scrambling to deal with that reality as are we.

The agenda for action and report of the Pew Health Professions Commission observed that there have been three eras in health and disease in the United States. The first, an outgrowth of the germ theory of the late 1800s, was characterized by the use of personal hygiene and sanitary measures to quell the great epidemics of infectious diseases. The second, derived from the widespread use of antibiotics after World War II and the development of modern therapeutics and biotechnology, has resulted in the successful treatment of many acute diseases. (I note parenthetically that most subject matter in most nursing programs belongs to this era.) And the third, current state, the commission noted, is marked by increases in chronic, degenerative diseases of lifestyle and aging.

We are here to take up the challenge of the third and present era while envisioning what the future holds for nursing practice and nursing education. We will be enriched and inspired by a faculty of extraordinary talents, experiences, and insight. I know you will not regret being here.

1

Gerontological Nursing Issues and Opportunities for Twenty-First Century "Not for the Weak of Heart: The Politics of Long-Term Care"

Sister Rosemary Donley

What is the political agenda of the aged and why are the politics of long-term care not for the faint of heart? I will begin by identifying some concerns of the aged: income security, protection of assets, health promotion, care during periods of illness or disability, and a peaceful death. What role can or should the government play in considering or advancing this agenda? What are the politics of aging?

INCOME SECURITY

Most elderly persons live on fixed incomes. This source of income is threatened by both inflation and low interest rates. While contemporary literature identifies single mothers and children as the poor of America (Select Committee on Children, Youth, and Families, 1985), the real value of the dollar earned by the elderly during their working years is threatened by periodic recessions and bad economic times. The aged can do little to remedy or control this situation. In addition, they are vulnerable when the price of a service or good they need (e.g., health care) rises faster than the rate of inflation. Given the stability of their incomes, most older persons are more threatened by greater health care deductibles, increases in copayments, and the rising costs of prescription drugs than people whose incomes increase each year. All things being equal, persons on fixed incomes may not choose services, as immunizations, which are not fully covered by their health insurance. Older persons are often misinformed about the benefits of the Medicare program and other health insurance programs. A significant number of older people also believe that Medicare will assist them with long-term care costs if they need these services ("Survey," 1987). In fact, only a small proportion of the nursing home bill (less than 1.5 percent) is covered by any form of insurance, public or private (Beck et al., 1990). The majority of long-term care costs are borne by residents of nursing homes and their families (Levit et al., 1991). Mindful of these factors, it is difficult to say whether the outcry, which resulted when recipients of Medicare realized that they would be required to pay more for catastrophic health care, was a vote against catastrophic care or a vote to protect their limited incomes from further erosion in a health care environment that cannot regulate its own costs (Hess, 1990; Rock, 1991).

PROTECTION OF ASSETS

When older persons own homes, they are at risk when the neighborhood changes because of urban disintegration or renewal. We are most familiar with older persons who are imprisoned in high rises or afraid to leave their homes because of a prevalent drug culture or violence in the neighborhoods (Special Committee on Aging, 1981). Improvement in neighborhoods, however, also has its costs (Szegedy-Maszak, 1988). This is especially true when the neighbors are not consulted by urban planners or real estate developers. In the 1960s, Jesuit sociologist Trafford Maher speaking to students at St. Louis University said poignantly, "Slums are home." Several years ago when the District of Columbia tried to reclaim some of the Rhode Island Avenue corridor from the damage it sustained in the riots which followed the slaying of Martin Luther King, Jr., an interesting article appeared in the *Washington Post*. One of the old timers who lived near Scott Circle recalled watching "them" move into her neighborhood. She said that she knew her days were numbered when a resident of a restored home on the circle wore a sable coat to walk a strange looking dog. While urban renewal may be good for the economy, wonderful for the tax base of the municipality, and pleasing to the eye, dramatic changes in property values may be a mixed blessing for the elderly (Cole, 1992). In the past several decades, many elderly persons who rented small apartments in New York City found that developers/owners envisioned office complexes and condominia in their neighborhoods. The poor and the elderly may not be able to pay taxes on reevaluated property; they may not be able to relocate or move on up to the East Side, like that TV couple, the Jeffersons. Most older persons cannot mobilize as did the German-born residents of the North Side of Pittsburgh who did not want Interstate-279 in their backyards or the Department of Transportation's bulldozers to fell St. Boniface Church. Although the people eventually lost their homes, the designation of St. Boniface as an historical monument saved their church. Some 30 years later as the residents aged, Interstate-279 was completed and connected Pittsburgh with the North Hills of Allegheny County. Its pathway, however, respected the placement of the old church.

Why is asset protection so important to the elderly? Those who work with the elderly describe a concern and even a preoccupation with money and possessions. My work with first-generation Americans who immigrated from the United Kingdom and Europe and settled in the greater Pittsburgh area leads me to propose a wish for independence from children and a desire to leave an "estate" as another explanation for these concerns. Future plans and dreams are seriously threatened by severe disability (notably, immobility, incontinence, or dementia) or the loss of caretakers (Perry & Butler, 1990). These losses are significant because they often trigger placement in nursing homes. With the annual costs of nursing homes approximating $30,000 a year (Beck et al., 1990), it is not surprising that ordinary people find that their personal resources and savings are soon depleted. In order to qualify for Medicaid, the older person must "spend down," sell the house, and reduce personal assets (Meltzer, 1988). Near the end of life, a person faces the frightening prospect of a loss of independence and wealth. As such, income security and asset protection influence the health concerns and choices of the aged and the politics of agenda building.

HEALTH PROMOTION

Our society and its health care system value treatment more than prevention of illness or primary care. The United States Chamber of

Commerce predicts that we will spend approximately 817 billion dollars for health care in 1992 (Kent, 1992). If 1992 is a typical year, most of the expenses for the elderly will occur during the last month of their lives and be directed to hospitals and physicians to pay for high technology medical interventions (Jahnigen & Binstock, 1991). While the lack of preventative services affects persons of every age, it is most significant for pregnant women, children, and older persons—the so-called vulnerable members of society. Regular visual and dental screening with appropriate followup can improve well-being for the elderly. Illnesses to which the elderly are at greater risk (e.g., cancer) can be detected and treated earlier if regular physical exams include screening for common cancers (breast, colon, cervical, prostate). Other illnesses (e.g., pneumonia and influenza) can be prevented or modified by immunizations. Chronic illnesses (e.g., diabetes and hypertension) can be managed by primary care, medication, exercise programs, and good nutrition. All these relatively inexpensive, low ticket technologies can be carried out in ambulatory settings or the home. Most of these health care services can be managed by nurses. By emphasizing health promotion as a health care service, I am not suggesting that people will live forever. I am saying, however, that some health care dollars should be redirected to primary care and preventative services to the elderly.

HEALTH CARE SERVICES

Any discussion about service delivery to the elderly should recognize the large, heterogeneous nature of this group. One of the difficulties of Medicare, for example, a program designed to finance acute health care of the elderly, stems from the diversity of this population. In the United States, we introduce another stratification and level of complexity because we administer health care entitlements separately from social security payments and other programs to address social needs (e.g., food, housing, transportation, and income support). While Medicare is handled in one bureaucracy, social security pension services are handled in another. Most older Americans, we must remember, receive these benefits. Eligibility for increased governmental assistance with housing, food, health benefits, or additional income is determined by a test of means and is managed by state welfare agencies. In the so-called welfare states of western Europe, pensioners receive more coordinated benefits. In contrast, we can argue that the elderly in America enjoy greater access to high-technology medical care than their western European compatriots. Although this argument is founded on current data, my point lies elsewhere: our valuing of choice and independence and our dislike of welfare make it difficult for the elderly to negotiate benefits. By separating health care from other social needs, America ignores the practical difficulty in distinguishing between the *medical* and the *social*. The isolation of a medical cause of illness says little about the treatment and care required for the afflicted person in his or her environment. Because our segregated bureaucracy does not allow older persons to easily mix and match comprehensive care services, they suffer needlessly. (In this light, I am amused by the phrase "managed care." We lack the structures to manage care. We can only manage health insurance benefits.) American elderly are also affected economically by the administration of their complex benefit programs. Sheils estimates that the administration of Medicare's copayment system alone costs 18 billion dollars a year (Gladwell, 1992). Economist Uwe Reinhardt says it this way: "Whatever the virtues of pluralistic health care may be, Americans should realize that these virtues are purchased at a very stiff price" (Joint Economic Committee, 1989).

No health care agenda for the elderly can overlook the fact that today 12 percent of the population in the United States (some 28 million people) is 65 or over; that 9 million Americans receive long-term care and that 2 of these 9 million people live in the nation's nursing homes (Beck et al., 1990). We anticipate that one in four people will be at least 65 years old by 2050 and that 20 percent of this population will be 85 years of age or over in that year (Joint Economic Committee, 1989). Because per capita personal health care expenditures are four times greater for persons over 65 (Joint Economic Committee, 1989), demographic concerns influence any agenda for the elderly.

No agenda for the elderly can ignore that our health care system is expensive, oriented to treatment of acute illness, and driven by an enthusiasm for high-technology medicine. Success and growth in any alternate delivery system, as community based care or home care, seem to be more dependent upon support from health financing plans than from serious measurements of care outcomes or consumer preference. To prove this point, note the development within the home care industry since the passage of the Prospective Payment Amendments of 1983.

Any serious reading of efforts to reform the health delivery system also reminds us that the current state of affairs gives a significant economic and personal advantage to the members of the American Medical Association and the American Hospital Association. Their power base would be altered significantly if the acute-care hospital played a less significant role in the coordination and delivery of care. In effect, their members would lose power and income if nurses, pharmacists, nutritionists, or social workers could authorize, provide, and bill insurers for care. During the last half of this century, the historical evolution of health policy reveals that powerful forces can be amassed to block even minor changes in delivery or payment systems. This evolution also shows how central the health care industry is to the American economy. Given the fact that change occurs incrementally at best, any change that affects the income and influence of powerful groups will be slow in being instituted and always begin at the margins.

A PEACEFUL DEATH

It has been some time since hospitals have thought of themselves as places of death (McMillan et al., 1990). Yet in American hospitals so oriented to cure and treatment the question of peaceful death has grown in importance. Most patients and their families expect that treatment will be successful. This hope has been fostered by decades of biomedical research, nourished by the American quest for perfection and the belief that action, in this case medical intervention, will solve all health problems.

Clinical decisions are complicated by the high technology readily available in the hospital environment. Although medicine has greatly improved its science, there is still ambiguity and a dimension of trial and error in clinical medicine. Most persons would want high-technology medicine if such treatment would assure a return to well being even with some level of disability. However, many persons would prefer no treatment to the burden of continued dependence on ventilators or existence in some vegetative state. That technological development has progressed more rapidly than the evaluation or assessment of its usefulness determines its limitations; the actual outcome of a technology is not always known when intervention begins. Yet the prevailing ethos in medicine and nursing encourages action. The clinical impulse here is to help or at least to try. There is another variable to the technological imperative as well. Physicians have been trained to think that their education, their relationship to the patient, and the patient's seeking of help give them the authority to act in the patient's best interest. Such paternalistic behavior has continued despite studies that have shown that most physicians do not know their patients' wishes (Bedell & Delbanco, 1984). Given these issues, it is realistic to say that an agenda for the aging will consider affordability, access, and quality of health care.

THE ISSUE OF COST

Long-term care touches policy makers' "cost control nerve" more deeply than other health issues because it is associated with nursing home care, the most expensive of the long-term care options and the only option with which the government has practical experience. Eighty percent of health care expenses for the elderly cover nursing home care (Joint Economic Committee, 1989). Policy makers fear that any expansion of the federal role in long-term care will trigger an increase in nursing home beds and encourage persons, currently cared for by family members, to enroll in government programs. Mechanic (1989) argues that the nursing home should not be the threshold for determining public responsibility for long-term care. Yet our government's long-term care policy is a gate keeping or rationing schema to limit the use of publicly supported nursing home beds. An aged person who lives alone and needs assistance with meal preparation, housekeeping, or personal care must find, coordinate, and pay for these services; qualify for services under the Older Americans Act or state welfare programs; or be admitted to a nursing home. There are no "social-bridge" programs for the middle class or the near poor to enable them to obtain and coordinate affordable support services in the community. The change in the nature of the family, the increased number of women in the workforce (society's historical caretakers or as Elaine Brody, 1981, expresses it, the women in the middle), and the growth in the number of aged persons, accentuate the gaps in service delivery for the aged (Minkler, 1990). The separateness of the health and social programs in the United States has also determined a situation where each year billions of federal dollars are spent for acute care for older persons without regard to their ability to pay. On the other hand, the federal government applies a poverty level means test to a network of social support services and long-term care services. As a result, the near poor and the middle class suffer; they are the uncounted, socially uninsured.

Obviously, a new vision of long-term care which removes nursing homes from center stage is needed. Unfortunately, the recommendations of the Pepper Commission (1990), which proposed three months of free nursing home care to all "severely disabled citizens without regard to age or income," did little but offer a health pork barrel as it fueled the fires of cost-containment advocates. It did nothing to advance a realistic long-term care agenda.

Yet all blame cannot be laid on the public sector. Private initiatives have been slow to develop, and the elder market has been surprisingly neglected by product developers other than the American Association of Retired Persons (AARP). Nurses have also been entrapped within medical parameters. Although their services have emphasized health education, education of caregivers, and home-based care, nurses have not taken leadership in adult day care, geriatric exercise and fitness centers, and consultation/referral agencies that specialize in long-term care. Nor have they lobbied builders' associations, producers of food, insurers' associations, makers of nutritional supplements, Chambers of Commerce, or the entertainment and hotel industries on behalf of the elderly. The tragic result of such inertia is that innovation in long-term care is very slow in the private sector and held hostage at the federal level by bills for Medicare and Medicaid. Political arguments about cost or first-dollar coverage ignore the major gap in the development of comprehensive long-term care services. Any agenda that seeks to advance the health and welfare of older persons must awaken private and public sensibilities and be played out in New York, Chicago, and Los Angeles, as well as in Washington, D.C.

POWER AND DOMINANCE

Why have comprehensive long-term care needs of the elderly been poorly served? Old age, disability, and chronic illness do not fit with America's emphasis on youth or with the high-tech curative mode of tertiary care systems. Consequently, the United States, which spends more than any of the 20 Organization for Economic Cooperation and Development (OECD) nations for its form of health care, ranks twentieth in infant mortality and places eighth in average life expectancy (Joint Economic Committee, 1989). Callahan's (1987) explanation for our failures in long-term care is more cynical. He argues that the current economic and political gains enjoyed by physicians, insurers, and health care administrators make them resist any impetus for change. The legitimation of providers by the entitlement programs has given physicians and institutions control of access to all health care resources and the ability to direct the flow of dollars within the system. If the health care system exists to benefit these providers, then the existing hierarchy is viable and balanced. If, however, the mission of the health care system is to assist the ill and vulnerable, the current configuration is a distortion of power. Anyone who advocates for a more just system of health care delivery comes face to face with human structures that promote dominance and control of resources, decisions, and money. Redistribution of power and a change in the delivery system will require a commitment to the common good and a return to more altruistic values. Without virtue, it is unlikely that physicians and health care administrators will welcome any initiative that threatens their power or income.

However, if the long-term care system could be reoriented, older persons would have the opportunity to elect primary, preventive, and support service and the burden and cost of treatment would be reduced. Disruption of the monopolies and oligopolies, enjoyed for over a quarter of a century, and blessed by Medicare, would free some of the dollars invested in acute care. It would also create the stimulus for market and quality tests of non-medical, support services to the aged. Until there is a real opportunity to test some of the innovations that have worked in local communities on a national scale, we will continue to argue about our inability to afford long-term care. While this debate goes on, the poor and the middle class will be held captive to societal inertia and a medical establishment power game.

BELIEFS ABOUT THE GOOD LIFE

Most recently, the federal government has intervened to assure patients more autonomy in the clinical decisions that effect them. Beginning on December 1, 1991, health agencies that accept Medicare funds must offer written information to adult patients about their rights: to accept or refuse treatment; to prepare a living will; and to appoint a durable power of attorney to represent their wishes should they become unable to do so (Hudson, 1991).

However, there is no reason to think that patients will be able to make more informed choices or anticipate outcomes better than their physicians. Patients are being asked to foresee a frightening personal situation—incompetence coupled with a serious physical condition that threatens their lives. A scenario can be envisaged: "Do you want the doctors and the nurses to try to save your life? Do you want them to try if the chances are good, average, less than average?" Another more problematic scenario sounds like this: "Do you want treatment to be continued if the treatment has ceased to be effective? Do you want new treatments in this situation? Do you realize that if nothing more is done or if treatment is stopped you will probably die?"

There are positive and negative dimensions to the Patient Self-Determination Amendments of 1990. On the positive side, patients will be consulted about their wishes. These consultations may occasion personal reflections on life and death or stimulate dialogues with family members. Nurses and doctors will have more confidence that they are acting in the patients' interests. Yet the ambiguity of the clinical situation will remain. In this new environment, physicians and nurses may also find that they are being asked to carry out therapeutic choices with which they do not agree. The new law spreads the risk of mistakes as well as the responsibility for choice.

It seems unlikely that the new federal regulations will anticipate all contingencies or overcome moral dissonance. Tristram Engelhardt (1991) labels postmodern decision makers as "moral strangers." He uses this term to describe situations where people, who have lost faith in reason or no longer share common beliefs or religious values, are asked to make very important clinical decisions.

> *I use the term* moral strangers *to signal the relationship people have to one another when they are involved in moral controversies and do not share a concrete moral vision that provides a basis for the resolution of the controversies . . . but instead reciprocally and incorrigibly (regard) each other's position as morally misguided and perhaps offensive* (pp. xiii, xiv).

The long-term care issues set before us raise political questions about cost, power, and ethics. Because the stakes are high, change will be tedious and resisted. No single group, regardless of its status, can wage the battle successfully. If nurses are to be part of the coalition for reform, they must lay aside specialty and organizational preferences and work with the public, the administration, the Congress, the business community, and other groups which seek reform of the health agenda. Many of these groups have more at risk than the medical or hospital establishment because the current arrangement affects profit margins and raises the cost of American products in world markets. Then too we are gearing up for a real election and health is back on the agenda again. The timing for our *united* intervention may just be right.

REFERENCES

Beck, M., Hager, M., Beachy, L., & Joseph, N. (1990, March 20). Be nice to your kids. *Newsweek,* 72–75.

Bedell, S. E., & Delbanco, T. L. (1984, April 26). Choices about cardiopulmonary resuscitation in the hospital: When do physicians talk with patients? *The New England Journal of Medicine, 310*(17), 1089–1093.

Brody, E. (1981, October). Women in the middle and family help to older people. *Gerontologist, 21,* 471–480.

Callahan, D. (1987). *Setting limits: Medical goals in an aging society.* New York: Simon & Schuster.

Cole, A. (1992, February/March). Property tax relief, tax reform grabs spotlight. *Modern Maturity, 35*(1), 12.

Engelhardt, H. T., Jr. (1991). *Bioethics and secular humanism: The search for a common morality.* London: SCM Press.

Gladwell, M. (1992, February 6). Reforming the health care systems: An American paradox. *Washington Post,* A25.

Hess, J. L. (1990, May 21). The catastrophic health care fiasco. *The Nation, 250,* 698–700.

Hudson, T. (1991, February 5). Hospitals work to provide advance directives information. *Hospitals, 65,* 26 + .

Jahnigen, D. W., & Binstock, R. H. (1991). Economic and clinical realities: Health care for elderly people. In R. H. Binstock & S. G. Post (Eds.), *Too old for health care? Controversies in medicine, law, economics, and ethics* (pp. 13–43). Baltimore: Johns Hopkins University Press.

Joint Economic Committee, Congress of the United States. (1989, October 2). *A staff report summarizing the hearings on "The future of health care in America." Prepared for the use of the subcommittee on education and health.* Washington, DC: U.S. Government Printing Office.

Kent, C. (Ed.). (1992, January 27). Perspectives. *Medicine & health* (Supplement).

Levit, K. R., Lazenby, H. C., Cowan, C. A., & Letsch, S. W. (1991). National health expenditures, 1990. *Health Care Financing Review, 13*(1), 29–54.

McMillan, A., Mentnech, R. M., Lubitz, J., McBean, A. M., & Russell, D. (1990). Trends and patterns in place of death for Medicare enrollees. *Health Care Financing Review, 12*(1), 1–7.

Mechanic, D. (1989, May). Health care and the elderly. *The Annals of the American Academy of Political and Social Science, 503,* 89–98.

Meltzer, J. W. (1988). Financing long-term care: A major obstacle to reform. In S. Sullivan & M. E. Lewin (Eds.), *The economics and ethics of long-term care and disability.* Washington, DC: American Enterprise Institute for Public Policy Research.

Minkler, M. (1990). Generational equity and public policy debate of quagmire or opportunity. In P. Homer & M. Hostein (Eds.), *A good old age?* (pp. 222–239). New York: Simon & Schuster.

Patient Self-Determination Act of 1990. Washington, DC: U.S. Government Printing Office.

Perry, D., & Butler, R. (1990). Aim not just for longer life but expanded "health span." In P. Homer & M. Holstein (Eds.), *A good old age?* (pp. 87–89). New York: Simon & Schuster.

Recommendations to the Congress by the Pepper Commission. (1990, March). *Access to health care and long-term care for all Americans.* Washington, DC: U.S. Government Printing Office.

Rock, A. (1991). The crushing cost of health care. *Ladies' Home Journal, 108,* 125–126.

Select Committee on Children, Youth, and Families, U.S. Congress. (1985). *Children and families in poverty: Beyond the statistics.* Washington, DC: U.S. Government Printing Office.

Special Committee on Aging, U.S. Senate Hearing. (1981). *Older Americans fighting the fear of crime.* Washington, DC: U.S. Government Printing Office.

Staff. (1987, November). Survey: Most older beneficiaries unsure of insurance coverage. *Geriatrics, 42*(11), 33.

Szegedy-Maszak, M. (1988, November 20). D. C. the other Washington. *New York Times Magazine,* 44–47.

2

Issues and Opportunities for the Twenty-First Century: The Search for a Definition of Quality in Long-Term Care Settings

Donna A. Peters

In 1892, only four out of every one hundred Americans made it past their sixty-fifth birthday. In 1992, the ratio is twelve in one hundred, and by the year 2030 one in every five Americans will be "old." Furthermore, the older old (the over-85 contingent) are the nation's fastest growing age group. Living to be 100 is still an achievement with the number of centenarians in the country at about 45,000. However, by the year 2080 they are expected to number 5 million (Margolis, 1990). These seniors are all at risk for chronic illness and functional impairment.

Unfortunately, the long-term care system of the United States, a system based on *affordability*, is not designed to meet these needs. Instead of a continuum from discharge planning in hospitals, to home care, nursing homes, or hospice care that serves the people it is intended to serve, there is a fragmented and disorganized system with people shuttled to the wrong level of care and many falling between the cracks (Mitchell, 1989).

In effect, the long-term care system is an industry offering a multitude of services to a heterogeneous population through an array of service agencies using a maze of payment mechanisms. Each payment mechanism has its own system of copayments and limits, and a blizzard of paperwork required to provide and maintain services. The fragmentation continues to get worse. For the professions involved, there is confusion and misunderstanding resulting in poor direction for future caregivers. For the providers involved, there is the question of mission and the burden of rework for staff that leads to burnout. For the patient, there is the problem of access.

To date, the only real response to such a fragmented system has been more government regulation. Yet this regulation has not even begun to deal with the definition and measurement of *quality*. In fact, federal regulation is still dealing with assuring minimum safety requirements (Mitchell, 1989).

The real issue of quality in long-term care is quality of life for the patient. Dealing with the subjectively perceived quality of life issue is extremely complicated. Who determines it? How is it measured? How does one reimburse for those services equitably? How does one measure which service provider is doing the most for the patient's quality of life (Schroeder, Somers, & Peters, 1992)? In a study by Slevin et al. (1988), 108 patients and their physicians completed the same rating scales for measuring anxiety, depression, and quality of life. The correlations between the two sets of scores were poor, suggesting that the doctors could not accurately determine what the patients felt and that an accurate measurement for quality of life must come from the patients themselves. Thus, any approach that is developed for determining quality in long-term care must involve the patient.

In this paper, then, I will briefly discuss quality assurance in long-term care as it currently exists, enumerate and describe additional key elements that need to be considered in defining quality for long-term care, and discuss the implementation of these elements into practice and the implication it has on education.

QUALITY ASSURANCE

The traditional approach to quality—constantly searching for and correcting negative experiences such as mistakes, incompetence, or harmful outcomes—rests in the assurance of its presence. Because negative experiences are believed to be caused by inadequate caregivers, solutions have centered on improving the caregiver's ability or removing the caregiver from the situation (Peters, 1992).

Such negative experiences are uncovered through the collection and measurement of data against defined standards. In this way, problems can be detected and the nurse or other caregivers can be told how to improve. As a result, assuring quality requires the establishment of extensive routine and systematic (often boring) data collection systems usually in the form of retrospective audits done by an outside quality assurance department or committee (the "quality police"). These audits include setting and measuring standards for each element of care provided by the organization. Quality is assured if all the standards are met, that is, if there are no negative experiences (Peters, 1991b).

Although this method is valuable, it does exhibit certain built-in limitations: (1) quality is only defined through the absence of negatives, never for what it represents; (2) information is usually incomplete or inaccurate because staff tend to hide or distort data to protect themselves from being found incompetent, thereby distorting the real picture; and (3) staff spend their energy on defending their ability or competence rather than improving their performance. Thus, the elusive *quality* is always trying to be assured by securing no negative findings on audits that were conducted using complete and accurate information. The cycle perpetuates, always hoping for better data next time. Even if quality is assured, the audits are always on yesterday's data, so it is impossible to know what is happening today (Peters, 1992).

Unfortunately, there is no quick fix to overcome these limitations. There are basic elements for quality in long-term care, however, that provide direction for successive steps, including: (1) get the client involved; (2) utilize a nursing model; (3) have a well-defined quality management plan; and (4) incorporate the use of outcomes.

KEY ELEMENTS FOR QUALITY

Redefining a quality system for long-term care must incorporate what clients want and need, their perceptions of their condition, and their expectations about what can be achieved through care. This means overcoming several current barriers: (1) the current fragmented system and its many nonintegrated quality assurance systems; (2) finding one set of quality standards to govern an entire plan of care regardless of agency or funding source; (3) addressing every aspect of care that affects the consumer; and (4) the conflict between the client's perception of what he or she needs and the provider's belief of what it can and should provide (Riley et al., 1989).

The Consumer

Involving the consumer will not only have a positive impact on the system; it will also impact on the consumer. In a study by Langer (1989), the effects of responsibility and decision making were explored on residents in a nursing home. The residents were divided into experimental and comparison groups. Residents in the experimental group were encouraged to make decisions for themselves. For example, they were asked to choose where they wanted to receive visitors—in their room, outdoors, in the dining room, lounge, or elsewhere; they were asked if they wanted to see a movie and, if so, to choose when they wanted to see it; they were given a house plant to care for and were to choose when and how much to water it, whether to put it in the sun or shade and so on. Conversely, residents in the comparison group were not encouraged to make any decisions, but were told that there was a very caring staff that would take care of them in every possible way. Residents in the comparison group were also given plants, but were told that the nurses would take care of them. Both groups were tested before and after the experiment using various behavioral and emotional measures to judge the effect of decision making. Consequent ratings showed a dramatic improvement for the experimental group—they had been given more of a chance to make decisions. Eighteen months later followup was done: the residents in the experimental group still took more initiative, were more active, vigorous, and sociable than residents in the control group. Even more impressive was the lower mortality rate seen in the experimental group. Before the study began, the health evaluation ratings for the two groups had been equivalent. Eighteen months later the health of the experimental group had improved and that of the comparison group worsened. Furthermore, only seven of the 47 persons in the experimental group died during the 18-month period, whereas 13 of the 44 persons in the comparison group had died (15 percent vs. 30 percent). The implication here is that taking care of someone (as in doing things for them) may in truth not be the best thing for them. It appears healthier for the client to be involved in his or her own life and life choices. The researcher for this particular study concludes that watching someone else do things that we used to do ourselves leads to feelings of incapability even if the inaction is a result of things outside of ourselves such as institutional policy.

Knowing that getting clients involved is therapeutic to their quality of life and knowing that physicians or nurses can't accurately measure a person's quality of life (Slevin et al., 1988) seem like solid reasoning for involving long-term care clients in their care and in evaluating the quality of that care. However, caregivers still find all the perfect reasons for not involving the consumer to a greater extent. Although these reasons are described elsewhere and at greater length in the literature (Peters, 1991a), I will summarize them here:

1. Difficulty in engaging the consumer because of personal barriers such as incoherence, coma, or poor hearing.
2. Caregivers' belief that they should determine the client's needs and that they should be determined by observation, not communication (Riley et al., 1989).
3. Consumers typically identify fewer needs than professionals do (due to undercommunication), but professionals develop care plans based on reimbursable services rather than on the needs of the client (Riley et al., 1989).
4. Consumers lack the information needed to make informed choices or to know what to ask.
5. The professional's assumption is that the quality of medical care is determined by the technical competence of the provider and that consumers are unable to evaluate technical competence. However, the majority of long-term care is not highly technical and, in addition, highly technical care that is being done in the home is often conducted by family members who have been trained.
6. Consumers are interested in quality of life, and health care is but a part of the concept of quality of life. Thus, most professional standards reflect only a part of the concept of quality of life. As such, it is time to consider quality measurements that link health care to quality of life, rather than continuing to link them to fragments of care such as skills or processes. Quality measurements then become the outcomes that include the preferences and expectations of the consumer.

Nursing Model

Federal regulations for long-term care continue to emphasize the medical need for care and the availability of skilled care and technical services. Such emphasis, however, is not true everywhere. For example, in England a nursing home is defined as a place where a qualified nurse is in charge. Regulations focus on nursing outcomes, such as maintaining an environment supportive of patient independence, rather than on medical indices. This distinction greatly influences the determination of quality. Again, in England, nursing homes do not use physical restraints whereas in the United States the prevalence of restraint use in similar institutions is almost 40 percent. Perhaps this is because in England patient falls are an accepted consequence of maintaining patient independence important to quality of life whereas in the United States they are a marker of poor care (Mezey, 1989).

If quality of life is the issue, then the more appropriate model for long-term care is a nursing model. Such a model considers the quality of the consumers' care in relationship to their values, family, and environment and not just their level of wellness. A healed wound, the range of blood sugars, or a fractured hip have significance only within the context of the greater whole. In establishing measurements of quality, therefore, values of both the caregiver and client should be examined. Covey (1990) indicates that, while values are the lens through which each of us view the world, most people are unaware of what their values are. Vance (1991) has determined three values of particular importance for the coming century: empowerment, caring, and cooperation. Although I have examined these values in greater depth elsewhere (Peters, 1992), I will review them here.

Empowerment. Empowerment is defined as having the authority to do what needs to be done to get the job done at that time. It is having the power "*to,*" not the power "*over.*" For example, the power "to" is the ability to take charge and get the family and client whatever help they need. The power "over" is doing it for the client and family without their knowledge, desire, or choice for what that help is. Allowing the client and family to make the choice empowers them in their own care. Staff and students can only empower their clients to establish and move toward realistic, attainable outcomes if they themselves are empowered. After all, it makes sense that staff and students will treat their clients similarly to the way they are treated; for example, if a student has to ask his or her instructor permission to render care, the student is more likely to have his or her clients call him or her to ask permission to call the physician rather than empowering them to act on their own. This concept of empowerment is especially important for the nurse in long-term care where the physician is absent and the nurse needs to function in isolation.

Caring. Caring is usually thought about as warm fuzzies with lots of tender loving care, as in "taking care of." However, "taking care of" we now know is not necessarily beneficial to the client. Caring encompasses the personal accountability that accompanies empowerment. For example, caring is being accountable to our clients by providing them all the information they need to make informed choices, presented in such a manner that the client has the best chance to understand the choice(s) available. Furthermore, once the client has made a choice, caring then becomes the professional's assessment, management, teaching, and provision of care required for the client to reach desired outcomes.

Caring, of course, is oriented to people and relates to quality through focusing on positive improvement in the person, whether that be physical, psychological, or both. One challenge in quality is to move past the "I gotcha" process; to move from the "You did it wrong" to the more caring approach of "How can we do it more effectively?" Such positive restructuring starts with what actually happened and moves toward the procurement of therapeutic results. For example, reconsider peer review (finding what you did wrong) as peer praise by acknowledging who you are, what you do well, and what opportunities for improvement exist.

Cooperation. When empowered and caring people work together toward a common goal in such a way that all are recognized and growth is encouraged, they are cooperating with each other. In this light, there is a potential in cooperation to enhance client outcomes. But this requires a collegial relationship with other peers, employees, clients, supervisors, and teachers rather than a hierarchical relationship. Such a collegial environment, however, rests on the establishment by those involved of new lines of communication and new ways of relating with each other with honesty, trust, and respect.

Cooperation can be encouraged in the following ways: (1) involving staff and/or students in decision making; (2) providing the opportunity for more informal communication among persons of different "levels" within the organization; (3) creating an environment that allows students/staff to admit their mistakes without fear of recrimination; (4) fostering creativity by holding contests and offering rewards; and (5) honestly and frequently praising people for what they do well.

Quality Management Plan

Moving beyond current limitations in assuring quality requires that quality be managed rather than assured. The components of managing quality need to be viewed within a philosophical context of long-term care and include a definition of quality, a defined mission, and a plan.

A definition for quality that includes the consumer and has a positive focus has been established for the home care industry through the "In Search of Excellence in Home Care" project. This $1.2 million project funded by the W.K. Kellogg Foundation to develop client-oriented outcomes for home health care incorporates client preferences for outcomes, the producer of the service or staff person, and the organization that provides the structure for the services. Their definition of quality reads: "The degree to which consumers progress toward desired outcomes, which they have established with the guidance and support of health care providers. These providers are part of an administratively and financially sound organization that maintains a competent staff and an environment encouraging personal excellence" (Peters, 1992).

Any discussion of quality management must include a look at the mission statement for the particular organization. It is in the mission statement that the values of the organization are articulated, and the direction for achievement and quality measurement determined. For example, what is the mission of a given extended care facility—is it a quasihospital, a short-term physical rehabilitation center, or a convalescent home? Although each of these are admirable missions, each will incorporate very different values and determinants of achievement and quality.

Finally, for managing quality there must be a plan. It is as important for the plan to reflect the organization's mission and beliefs about long-term care as it is for all those concerned to be involved in the development and execution of the plan. In this sense, involvement in and responsibility for quality care are shared equally. Also inherent in a successful plan is a concurrent system for data collection and analysis. In fact, the more that data collection can be incorporated into people's daily routines, the more efficient the process and the greater the chances for accurate and complete information.

A quality management plan consists of the key areas that a given organization views as important to monitor in determining quality. In a convalescent home, for example, a key element or pulse point might be human relationships—the bond between nurse and patient. Places to look for ideas for pulse points include the organization's mission statement, new programs, or those areas that have been problematic in the past such as deficiencies in state or federal surveys. For each pulse point as well there should be at least one outcome that will indicate whether or not a problem exists. For each outcome, a person needs to be identified as responsible for collecting the data, defining from what source the data will be obtained, and how often the data will be changed to information (usually by adding the denominator) and reviewed to determine trends. The layout would look like this:

Quality Management Plan (Peters, 1992)

Pulse points	Outcomes	Source	Reviewer	Frequency

The plan should be reviewed in its entirety at least annually to determine what pulse points (if any) and accompanying measurements should be added or deleted. If a given outcome measurement has been at a consistent level that is considered "quality" for the organization for a year, it is probably satisfactory to drop it. However, it should be noted that exceptional achievement on a given outcome is excellent marketing material and thus continued measurement may be warranted. It should also be remembered that a successful plan will only measure those *key* areas for quality and not necessarily quantity (as in measuring everything). A successful implementation of a plan will start slowly, perhaps with just one pulse point. Ideally, the first pulse point chosen will be an easy one that will be successfully implemented, thereby encouraging behavior that is satisfying for staff. Unfortunately, all too often organizations choose the most difficult pulse points first and then get discouraged when success is not immediate.

Outcomes

Since long-term care has been molded by a medical model with an institutional bias, the quality assurance system has been limited to the "institution," where the client is a patient, and focused on getting the patient "better." "Better" has been broadly defined to include peaceful death for the terminally ill, especially in hospice care. However, for quality to exist in long-term care, the consumers and their expectations of service (outcome) must be considered as well as the care rendered by the caregiver (process) and the organization(s) providing the care (structure). Outcomes focus on the results of service delivery. They determine how a service affects the client's well-being (Wennberg, 1991). Since the goal of long-term care is quality of life, outcomes need to consider the patient's environment and social, cultural, emotional, and spiritual situation, not just a "healed wound." This notion of consumer outcomes is still in its infancy.

Three levels of consumer outcomes need to be considered (Peters & Eigsti, 1991), with each level used separately or interactively to complement each other: individual, intra-organizational, and inter-organizational. For each level, the outcome becomes a benchmark to evaluate movement toward the desired end. The individual level (used as a part of care plans) measures client progress, the intra-organizational level (used in quality management plans) measures agency quality or progress toward their mission, and the inter-organizational level (largely nonexistent right now) measures industry quality by allowing inter-organizational comparisons.

The key elements to an outcome are: (1) it includes the client's choice for quality of life and is philosophically aligned with a nursing model; (2) it is determined in response to a client or agency "problem" (e.g., a client's nursing diagnosis or organizational pulse point); (3) it contains a measurable expected behavior; and (4) it includes a time frame measured in either days (weeks, months) or visits (i.e., at what point it is estimated that this behavior will take place). An example of an individual outcome follows: Mr. Jones will put on his own shirt and pants without assistance in one week. An example of an intra-organizational outcome is: All patients will be free of signs and symptoms of infection three weeks after admission. Inter-organizational outcomes would be similar to the intra-organizational outcomes except they would be measured across organizations.

IMPLEMENTATION INTO PRACTICE

Work is now underway in implementing the concepts just discussed. The "In Search of Excellence in Home Care" project, for example, has included the consumer in defining home care quality and has incorporated a holistic approach (e.g., consumers viewed within the context of their environment, and so on). Quality of care and quality of life is determined by what the consumers want and whether they get what they wanted.

The goal of the project is to strengthen the home care industry by developing consumer-oriented outcomes that will allow for interagency comparisons. The project is divided into four major phases: (1) design and development, which includes a literature review and the use of consumer focus groups and other advisory bodies and reports; (2) operationalization, which includes a short pilot and then concurrent data collection utilizing the instruments at nine data collection sites across the country; (3) evaluation, which includes completion of data collection and analysis; and (4) integration of the findings into the Community Health Accreditation Program (CHAP) process on a more concurrent basis. CHAP is a voluntary accreditation organization that has been accrediting community health organizations since 1965.

The project developed a home care industry quality management plan. There are 11 pulse points, divided into three categories: the consumer, clinical, and organizational. For each pulse point, an outcome, a data collection instrument, an accountable person, and a time frame was defined.

A total of seven data collection instruments were designed. Two Likert scale survey instruments were developed to measure the five consumer based outcomes—one administered within two weeks of admission and the second administered within two weeks of discharge. To measure clinical outcomes, there is a clinical assessment form consisting of 18 functional items and 16 physiological items that is also completed at patient admission and discharge. For each item the consumer is asked to describe expected outcomes. There is an additional measurement using the first clinical instrument which takes place if the patient is still in care after 45 days. Survey tools were also developed to assess the quality of health care by staff members and administration (organizational outcomes) which are completed once during the term of the project. Finally, an agency data form was developed to obtain organizational data compiled during the year.

Although data collection will not be completed until the end of the year and quantitative data not available until after that, several interesting observations have come forth. For example, many staff asked questions about how to ask clients what they want, implying that the clients had not really been involved as "partners" in care before. In addition, roughly 30 percent of clients eligible to participate in the project refused. In investigating these refusals, it was discovered that some clients were never asked and that it was the nurse's arbitrary determination that the client not participate.

Many of these scenarios can be attributed to uncertainty and discomfort on the part of staff, as well as to barriers in the current system. What is exciting here, however, is a noticeable behavior change in staff as they have had an opportunity to participate and their discomfort is reduced. Furthermore, as the project continues, the agencies are empowering staff more by reducing some of the barriers to implementation of the full project. For example, one main barrier is that of staff having to maintain productivity levels while doing the extra work required by the project. Agencies have dealt with this in various ways such as (1) streamlining admission procedure for project participants, (2) reducing productivity demands on staff with project participants in their caseload, and (3) directly reimbursing staff for the extra project work.

In any event, the project is showing that although there is initial discomfort with this new approach to quality, the opportunity for trying new approaches in a safe environment (as part of a study), continued support from experts, and persistent encouragement over time allows for growth and integration of the concepts.

IMPLICATIONS FOR EDUCATION

Because quality in long-term care is expanded to consider quality of life and not just health care, student skill ranges require some reorientation. For example, students need to be aware of sociological factors and the role of ethical, sociopsychological, psychological, and cultural attitudes of the client and family toward well-being (Smith, 1988).

Furthermore, with the greater inclusion of the clients in their care, students need the opportunity to reexamine the nurse–client relationship. The nurses' role becomes more of educator and facilitator of client choices. Ethical dilemmas of what to do if the client's choice differs from that of the nurse and the nurse is placed into a position of implementing a care plan with which he or she doesn't agree to must also be examined.

Students use their learning experience as a model. For students to be more comfortable in a collegial relationship with clients as well as with other team members, they need a more collegial relationship with faculty. This can be facilitated with the use of more active participatory learning strategies such as writing and group discussions.

Attitude is another area for consideration. Attitudes toward the values of empowerment, caring, and cooperation need to be examined and old beliefs like those mentioned earlier need to be discussed and discarded. Attitudes toward quality also need to be reexamined. Quality needs to be internalized as something everyone participates in all the time. A mistake should be welcomed as an opportunity for quality rather than covered over as an embarrassment. Mistakes show us what we need to learn. Covey (1989) states that not acknowledging a mistake, correcting it, and learning from it is another mistake. This coverup mistake puts a person on a self-deceiving, self-justifying path that involves rational lies to oneself and others. John Roger and Peter McWilliams (1991) describe the process of learning in this fashion: (1) act, (2) look for mistakes, (3) figure out how to do it better next time, and (4) act.

Finally, the notion of using outcomes needs to be reincorporated into the learning process. While outcomes resemble "behavioral objectives" in many ways, they need to be made less academic and more real. Students can be encouraged to establish their own outcomes for their own learnings for a given course, assignment, or whatever. The more comfortable they are with outcomes, the easier it will be for them to assist their clients in determining outcomes for care. And the less threatening it will be for them to establish outcomes within their place of employment for determining and monitoring quality.

America is aging and requiring more use of a long-term care system. The current system falls short of meeting their needs. Measuring quality in this system also suffers from the limitations of the system. Expanding the definition of quality and how it is approached may be a beginning to changing the whole system. Thus, this article has outlined some of the issues and opportunities before us as the twenty-first century approaches.

REFERENCES

Covey, S. R. (1990). *The seven habits of highly effective people.* New York: Simon & Schuster.
Roger, J., & McWilliams, P. (1991). *Do it.* Los Angeles: Prelude Press.
Langer, E. J. (1989). *Mindfulness.* Addison-Wesley.
Margolis, R. J. (1990). *Risking old age in America.* Boulder: Westview Press, Inc.
Mezey, M. (1989). Institutional care: Caregivers and quality. In *Indices of quality in long-term care: Research and practice* (pp. 155–169). New York: National League for Nursing.
Mitchell, M. K. (1989). Long-term care. In *Indices of quality in long-term care: Research and practice* (pp. 1–5). New York: National League for Nursing.
Peters, D. A. (1991a). Consumer oriented quality assurance in home care. *Pride Institute Journal, 10*(2), 8–13.
Peters, D. A. (1991b). Measuring quality: Inspection or opportunity? *Holistic Nursing Practice, 5*(3), 1–7.

Peters, D. A. (1992). A new look for quality in home care. *Journal of Nursing Administration*.

Peters, D. A., & Eigsti, D. M. (1991). Utilizing outcomes in home care. *Caring, 10*(10), 44–45.

Riley, T., Colburn, A., Fortensky, R., & Palmer, M. (1989). *Developing consumer centered quality assurance strategies for home care*. University of Southern Maine, Human Services Development Institute.

Schroeder, S., Somers, S., & Peters, D. (1992). *Home care in America*. Presentation prepared for University of Florida Forum for Health Care.

Slevin, M. L., Plant, M., Lynch, D., Drinkwater, J., & Gregory, W. M. (1988). Who should measure quality of life, the doctor or patient? *British Journal of Cancer, 57*, 109–112.

Smith, J. B. (1988). Public health and the quality of life. *Family Community Health, 10*(4), 49–57.

Vance, M. (1991). Management by values seminar. National Association of Home Care, MA.

Wennberg, J. E. (1991). A patient outcomes orientation: a response. In M. S. Donaldson, J. Harus-Wehling, & K. L. Lohr (Eds.), *Medicare: New director in quality assurance*. Washington, DC: National Academy Press.

3

New Practice Models in Long-Term Care

*Christine Heine and
Sister Rose Therese Bahr*

Where will gerontological nurses be practicing in the twenty-first century? What types of practice models will be used by gerontological nurses to provide services to elderly clients? What should nurse educators and administrators do to prepare current and future nurses for these different settings and practice models? In this chapter, we will briefly evaluate demographic projections related to long-term care, summarize three key documents on the future of health care, and examine several successful models for providing nursing services in long-term care. We will conclude with twelve predictions for the future of gerontological nursing within the context of future practice settings and practice models.

WHO NEEDS LONG-TERM CARE NOW? WHO NEEDS IT IN THE FUTURE?

In September 1990, the Pepper Commission, a bipartisan commission on comprehensive health care, submitted their final report recommending how to ensure that all Americans had coverage for health care and long-term care.* The Pepper Commission defined long-term care as an array of services needed by individuals who have lost some capacity for independence because of a chronic illness or condition. It consists of assistance with basic activities and routines of daily living and may also include skilled and therapeutic care for the treatment and management of chronic conditions. Long-term care services can be provided in a variety of settings—the individual's home, the community, or an institution.

Between 9 and 11 million Americans of all ages (1 in 20) need assistance with one or more activities of daily living (ADL) or independent activities of daily living (IADL). Two-thirds of the long-term care population are elderly persons living in the community or nursing homes. One quarter of the nation's elderly population (seven million) are limited in ADLs and IADLs. By the year 2030, almost 14 million elderly persons in the community will require assistance with activities of daily living (The Pepper Commission, 1990).

WHERE DO PEOPLE LIVE THAT NEED LONG-TERM CARE?

Almost 9 million people of all ages who need long-term care live in the community compared to less than 2 million persons that live in an institutional setting. Fifty-nine percent of the severely disabled live at home (The Pepper Commission, 1990).

The primary users of nursing homes are those persons over 65 years. Nine out of 10 nursing home residents are elderly and almost half are over the age of 85. Among people turning age 65 in 1990, estimates are that 36 to 45 percent will use a nursing home before they die; however, at any given day, 5 percent of elderly persons are in nursing homes. Women have a much higher risk than men for residing in a nursing home. More than half are likely to spend time in a nursing home compared with only one-third of men (The Pepper Commission, 1990).

---

* Statistics about long-term care are taken from *The Pepper Commission Report*, September, 1990.

HOW DO PEOPLE GET LONG-TERM CARE AND PAY FOR IT?

In 1988, $53 billion was spent on long-term care, but only 18 percent went to home care despite the fact that four out of five disabled and almost three out of five severely disabled live at home. The great majority of long-term care in the home is provided by families and friends, but not without enormous physical, financial, and emotional cost. When families want to purchase care, they may have trouble finding it and must bear its full cost. There are very few public programs that provide long-term care services in the home or community. Approximately 75 percent of elderly persons who were severely disabled and receiving long-term care at home or in the community in 1989 relied solely on family members or other unpaid help (The Pepper Commission, 1990).

Nursing home care is highly subsidized by public funds. Total spending on nursing home care is split about evenly between the public and private sectors.

More than 7 million spouses, adult children, other relatives, friends, and neighbors provided unpaid assistance to disabled elders. Seven out of 10 informal caregivers bear the major responsibility for the care of disabled elders and one of three is a sole provider. Care provided averages four hours a day, seven days a week. The great majority of the caregivers are female and 35 percent of them are 65 years and older (The Pepper Commission, 1990).

These telling statistics support three important reports or documents recently published that provide insight into determining long-term care services for older persons as well as practice models that will be needed for providing these services. The Pew Health Professions Commission released a report entitled *Healthy America: Practitioners for 2005*. This report projects competencies that will be required by health care professionals by the year 2005 to meet people's health care needs. Through careful analysis of demographic, economic, and health care data, the Pew Commission proposed 17 competencies required of health care practitioners in the year 2005. Most of these competencies are directly applicable to gerontological nursing. Table 1 provides an overview of these competencies and their relevance to gerontological nursing. These competencies are designed to be used by universities with schools for health professionals. In addition to developing these competencies for health care professionals, America will require more health professionals to address the needs of older adults.

Table 1
Competencies for Health Care Practitioners* and Relevance to Gerontological Nursing

Competencies from Commission*	Relevance to Gerontological Nursing
Care for community's health through broad understanding of the determinants of health.	Determinants of healthy aging.
Expand access to effective care.	Access to health care for older individuals.
Provide contemporary clinical care by possessing up-to-date clinical skills.	Skills in functional and mental status assessment, environmental assessment; knowledge about effect of relocation, loss, and grieving.
Emphasize primary care and able to function in new health care settings.	Primary care in senior housing, community centers, and shopping centers.
Participate in coordinated care by working effectively as team members of an interdisciplinary team.	Discharge planning for older adults.
Ensure cost-effective and appropriate care by balancing cost and quality in the decision-making process.	Knowledge about Medicare, Medicaid, Medigap coverage.
Emphasize primary and secondary preventive strategies for all people.	Preventive health care practices specific to health risks for older adults.
Involve patients and families in the decisions regarding personal health care and in evaluating its quality and acceptability.	Self-responsibility for health and health care; i.e., living will, support groups, appeal process for denial of health care payment; identifying health care providers accepting assignment.
Promote healthy lifestyle.	Strategies and information for maintaining health while aging.
Assess and use technology appropriately.	Effectiveness of technology for older adults.
Improve the health care system and be knowledgeable about the system from a broad political, economic, social, and legal perspective.	Nuances of the long-term care system. Coordination efforts to improve access and accountability.

Table 1 *(Continued)*

Competencies from Commission*	Relevance to Gerontological Nursing
Manage and use large volumes of scientific, technological, and patient information.	Information systems for storing, retrieving, and sharing information about elderly clients; access information about appropriate care for elderly clients.
Understand the role of the physical environment.	Fall prevention, automobile safety for older adults, hypo and hyperthermia risks.
Provide counseling on ethical issues.	Withdrawal of nutritional and respiratory support; power-of-attorney; competency laws.
Responsive to increasing levels of public, governmental, and third-party participation in the shape and direction of the health care system.	Expansion of coverage for long-term care; health care reform.
Appreciate the growing racial and cultural diversity of the population.	Health care needs and practices of older adults of different races and cultures.
Anticipate changes in health care and respond by redefining and maintaining professional competency throughout practice life.	Certification in gerontological nursing; continuing education to maintain competence in gerontological nursing.

* *Source:* Pew Health Professions Commission, *Healthy America: Practitioners for 2005.* 1991. Durham, N.C.

A second report, *Healthy People 2000: National Health Promotion and Disease Prevention Objectives,* is a national initiative sponsored by the U.S. Public Health Service which forwards objectives to ensure a healthier public and targets a variety of age groups, including older adults (Office of Disease Prevention and Health Promotion, 1990). Improving the functional independence, not just the length, of later life is an important element in promoting the health of older adults. A growing body of evidence shows that changing certain health behaviors, even in old age, can benefit health and quality of life. A key ingredient to healthy aging is physical activity. A major result of regular physical activity appears to be the maintenance of functional independence throughout the later years of life (Office of Disease Prevention and Health Promotion, 1990).

Primary health care services are needed by older adults to help maintain health and prevent disabling and life-threatening diseases and conditions. Thus, clinical preventive services include the control of high blood pressure, screening for cancers (mammography and breast exams), immunization against pneumonia and influenza, counseling to promote healthy behaviors (proper medication use, keeping an active mind and intellect), and therapies to help manage chronic conditions such as arthritis, osteoporosis, and incontinence. In addition, community support networks that provide services to help older adults maintain independence are critical interventions for reducing social isolation. Many older adults are at risk for social isolation. Depression is a frequent outcome of the life changes common in the seventh and eighth decades that can increase the risk of social isolation. Men aged 65 through 74 have the highest suicide rate in the United States (Office of Disease Prevention and Health Promotion, 1990).

Key *Healthy People 2000* objectives have been targeted for improving the health of older adults. A summary of these objectives is provided in Table 2.

Nursing's Agenda for Health Care Reform, spearheaded by the American Nurses' Association and the National League for Nursing in 1991, is the third document that can help determine future practice settings and models for the care of older adults. This document proposes a plan to

Table 2
Summary of National Health Objectives Targeting Old Adults from Healthy People 2000[*]

1. Reduce suicides among white men aged 65 and older.
2. Reduce deaths caused by motor vehicle crashes.
3. Reduce deaths from falls and fall-related injuries.
4. Reduce residential fire deaths.
5. Reduce hip fractures.
6. Reduce the proportion of people who have lost all of their natural teeth.
7. Increase years of healthy life to at least 65 years.
8. Reduce the proportion of persons who have difficulty in performing two or more personal care activities, thereby preserving independence.
9. Reduce significant hearing impairments.
10. Reduce significant visual impairments.
11. Reduce epidemic-related pneumonia and influenza deaths.

[*] *Source:* U.S. Department of Health and Human Services, Public Health Service, Office of Disease Prevention and Health Promotion. *Healthy People 2000: National Health Promotion and Disease Prevention Objectives.* 1990. Publication No. 017-001-00473.

reform the health care system ensuring access to health care, quality health care, and cost-effective health care for all Americans. The restructured health care system proposed includes the following:

1. Enhances consumer access to services by delivering primary health care in community-based settings.
2. Fosters consumer responsibility for personal health, self-care, and informed decision making in selecting health care services.
3. Facilitates utilization of the most cost-effective providers and therapeutic options in the most appropriate settings (American Nurses Association, 1991).

Included in the plan is a key aspect for health care reform: the delivery of primary health care services to households and individuals in convenient, familiar places. The rationale used to support the delivery of such care is clear. If health is to be a true national priority, it is logical to provide services in the places where people work and live (American Nurses' Association, 1991).

NEW PRACTICE MODELS

In the last several years, nurses have successfully developed and implemented practice models that are responsive to the health care needs and living situations of older adults. Brief descriptions of several new practice models follow.

EverCare, developed by two nurses employed by a Health Maintenance Organization (HMO) in Minnesota, provides health care services to nursing home residents that are members of the HMO. Services are provided by geriatric nurse practitioners and geriatricians (Polich et al., 1990). Another example, also in Minnesota, is the block nurse program that provides services to keep older persons in their homes with case management by public health nurses living in the community (Jamison, Campbell, & Clark, 1989).

The On Lok Senior Health Service program has been one of the most successful comprehensive long-term care programs in the country. The full range of social and medical services are planned and provided through a multidisciplinary team using a consolidated model of case management. The services are community based and provided to older persons that are determined appropriate for institutional care. Services are provided in a community center and in the home and include day care, meals, transportation, nursing and medical care, personal care, social services, rehabilitation services, homemaker, and chore services (Zawadski & Eng, 1988).

A number of nurse-managed health clinics at senior housing sites also exist. For example, there is a nurse-managed clinic provided in four mid-rise apartments owned and operated by the Norfolk Redevelopment and Housing Authority in Norfolk, Virginia. Through a grant from the Division of Nursing, U.S. Department of Health and Human Services, and in collaboration with Old Dominion University School of Nursing, the city of Norfolk was able to employ a full-time gerontological nurse practitioner (GNP) to provide a variety of health and health promotion services to older adults. The GNP recorded 532 visits to the clinics in the first five months of operation. The setting is also used as a clinical site for nursing students from the university (Heine, 1992).

These successful practice models, the demographic trends, and three documents reviewed all point to an exciting future for gerontological nursing. Gerontological nurses have many opportunities to develop new practice models and settings in response to the unique health care needs of older adults. We have proposed 12 predictions for gerontological nursing that are based on the data presented in this chapter. Readers are encouraged to use these predictions for determining new practice settings and models.

1. The practice of gerontological nursing will take place where older persons live, specifically their homes and housing designed for older adults.
2. The practice of gerontological nursing in long-term care nursing facilities will be a subspecialty requiring more professional nurses to provide, direct, and evaluate care to the ever increasing number of persons needing nursing home care.
3. Health promotion for older adults will be a major emphasis in the practice of gerontological nursing. Gerontological nurses will specialize in primary care.
4. Geropsychiatric nurses will be in demand both in the community and in long-term care nursing facilities.
5. Innovative programs and services will be developed and provided by gerontological nurses to support family members who are caregivers to older family members.

6. Acute-care hospitals will have at least one GNS on staff. Gerontological nursing subspecialties preferred for acute-care facilities will include critical care, trauma, oncology, rehabilitation, medical-surgical, opthamology, and psychiatry.
7. Gerontological nurses will be sought after by architectural firms, leisure service providers, medical product companies, and furniture companies to provide consultation on the development of environments, services, and products for older persons.
8. Individual physicians, large physician group practices, and coordinated care systems (HMOs, PPOs) will seek to employ nurses with background and expertise in care of older adults.
9. Gerontological nurses will be experts in case management, as defined in the community and in institutional settings.
10. Gerontological nurses will be competent and skillful in counseling older adults and their families in situations where ethical issues arise, as well as participate in discussions of ethical issues in health care as they affect older adults.
11. Gerontological nurses will develop and provide innovative services to older adults from culturally diverse backgrounds.
12. Gerontological nurses will be instrumental in developing policy that affects the health and well-being of older adults at the local, state, and national level.

These predictions provide challenges to nurse educators and nurse administrators in preparing current and future nurses to meet the health care needs of older adults. Current curricula in undergraduate and graduate programs need to be carefully scrutinized as well to ensure that students are knowledgeable and skilled in caring for older adults in a variety of settings and in various states of health. Practicing professional nurses require additional education and skill development in working with older adults.

Innovative care models for providing health services to older adults need to be promoted and supported by the nursing community. These models can be developed in settings where nurses already work (e.g., clinics, hospitals, nursing homes, home health, adult day care centers) with support of the institution or in new settings such as senior housing, community centers, churches, and schools. Care models specific to racially and culturally diverse older adults need to be developed.

Information, referral, coordination, and support programs responsive to family caregivers are needed. Nurses must take leadership roles in developing new care models in nursing homes and complementary programs and services between the community and the nursing home. Lobbying of state and federal legislators to reimburse gerontological nurses in advanced practice for their services in alternative settings other than institutions must continue. Finally, research is needed to identify the outcomes associated with new nursing practice models for the provision of health care to older adults.

REFERENCES

American Nurses' Association. (1991). *Nursing's agenda for health care reform*. Washington, DC: The Author.

Heine, C. (1992). *Model gerontological clinical sites project*. Final report to Division of Nursing, U.S. Department of Health and Human Resources. Grant #1D10 NU60064, Norfolk, VA: Old Dominion University.

Jamison, M., Campbell, J., & Clark, S. (1989). The block nurse program. *Gerontologist, 29*(1), 124–128.

Office of Disease Prevention and Health Promotion. (1990). *Healthy people 2000: National health promotion and disease prevention objectives*. U.S. Public Health Service. Pub. No. 017-001-00473. Washington, DC: U.S. Government Printing Office.

Pepper Commission. (1990, September). *A call for action*. Pub. No. S. Prt. 101-114. Washington, DC: U.S. Government Printing Office.

Pew Health Professions Commission. (1991). *Healthy America: Practitioners for 2005*. Durham, NC: Pew Commission.

Polich, C., Bayard, J., Jacobson, R., & Parker, M. (1990). A nurse-run business to improve health care for nursing home residents. *Nursing Economics, 8*(2), 96–101.

Zawadski, R., & Eng, C. (1988). Case management in capitated long-term care. *Health Care Financing Review* (annual supplement), 75–81.

4

The Nursing Home Clinical: New Horizons for Capitalizing on a Caring Experience

M. Elaine Tagliareni

Olin Peterson is 82 years old. For the past six months he has been returning to the hospital at regular intervals for chemotherapy. He is known by everyone. To each person who enters his room, bringing IV infusion pumps, more tubing, and vials of medications, he repeats the same request, "Excuse me nurse, did I tell you yet, I have to be home by 4:00. Excuse me nurse, I'll be home by 4:00, won't I?"

Anna Starkey is 87 years old. She is in the coronary care unit (CCU) of a large inner city hospital with another episode of congestive heart failure. She has lived in a nursing home for the past six years now; it's her home. As the nurse enters to check her A line and monitor her vital signs, she asks anxiously, "Excuse me nurse, can you tell me—Do I live here? Where is my apartment? Is this my room?"

Questions, simple requests really, powerful messages for nursing and for nursing practice in 1992: "Excuse me nurse, but do you know me? Do you understand me?"

I met Olin when he was a patient in an acute-care hospital, in the bed next to my father. He told me that he needed to be home by 4:00 because his daughter left for work and she helped him prepare for the night, setting up his bedtime routine. "If I'm late I'll be on my own," he said sadly. "And I don't do so well." When he left that day, at 5:00, he looked at me with resignation in his eyes and said, "Thanks for listening to me, nice lady—maybe I'll make it on time next week."

I met Anna when I was a faculty member in the nursing home. I came to know Anna, really love Anna, through the caring and thoughtful practice of a nursing student named Sarah. One morning, during a clinical rotation in the nursing home, Sarah stood by the elevator waiting for me to arrive. Sarah greeted me saying, "It's the third week of this rotation and I'm getting nowhere with Anna. All she ever says is, 'Do I live here? Is this my room? Where is my apartment? I am so discouraged."

Sarah and I went to talk with Anna. Together we conducted a thorough assessment and brainstormed about creative approaches to help Anna become more involved in daily activities at the nursing home. While conducting the interview, Sarah began to realize that Anna was less cognitively impaired than she had suspected at first and suggested that maybe Anna could manage quiet group events. Sarah was beginning to see Anna differently. That day in the nursing home, the group was playing Trivial Pursuit. As Sarah and Anna entered the dayroom, the group leader called out, "Oh, here is Sarah! Let's ask her a question. What is the longest river in the United States?" Sarah answered immediately, "Why it's the Mississippi, isn't it?" Standing next to her, Anna quietly murmured, "No, dear, it's the Missouri." At that moment, Sarah saw Anna differently.

The following week, Sarah arrived to find that Anna had been transferred to the coronary care unit of a local acute-care hospital. Sarah called the CCU nurse and asked about Anna. The nurse told Sarah all about Anna's blood studies, oxygen saturation, and cardiac status. Sarah asked again, "But how is Anna?" The CCU nurse said, "How would I know? All she ever says is, 'Do I live here? Is this my room? Where is my apartment?'" As she ended the conversation, Sarah said to the CCU nurse, "You would be surprised how much Anna really knows."

Later that day, Sarah came to talk to me. She had been thinking all day about her conversation with the CCU nurse. "I now know what I wanted to say to that CCU nurse. I wanted to say, 'Do you know the longest river in the United States? Anna does.' I wanted to say to that nurse, 'Go ahead and ask her; it will make all the difference. I know it did for me.'"

Knowing Olin and Anna and Sarah has made all the difference for me too. For those of us who have had the opportunity and privilege to be involved in the Community College–Nursing Home Partnership, their stories tell our story. It is a story about individuals—the Olins, the

Annas, the Sarahs in our lives who have changed our perspective on nursing. These individuals have refocused our thinking about nursing, about teaching nursing, and about nursing practice with older adults in a world, seized by technology, where the focus is on disease and its prevention and cure, where services are fragmented, where individuals like Olin and Anna so often become dehumanized. "Excuse me nurse, but do you know me?"

And ours is a story about the nursing home, a setting that project faculty have learned to appreciate and value, a setting where quality of life issues predominate. It is a setting where the focus is on health promotion and maintenance of optimal functional ability, on seeking rehabilitation potentials despite tremendous odds, a setting where the emphasis is on care and not cure.

In four years of working with students in the nursing home, partnership faculty have made a startling discovery. The nursing home is a unique setting, with its own culture and its own institutional ethic, its own nursing practice patterns. It is not the hospital! Because of that, the nursing home may very well be the best place to teach selected nursing concepts essential to nursing practice in all settings. Let me explain. We work today in a health care system where cure-oriented interventions and disease treatment modalities may, in fact, shortchange the growing numbers of older adults with multiple chronic illnesses and functional and cognitive disabilities, individuals like Olin and Anna, who require our care and support.

We teach nursing today in a world of very ill patients and rapid technological advances. This is a world characterized by complexity, ambiguity, and uncertainty. Within this context, nurse educators struggle continually to help students to think critically and creatively about clinical situations, to individualize nursing care, and, more specifically, to see the older adult as an individual with potential for growth and improved quality of life. Yet it is not easy. Last spring I walked by the office of one of my colleagues at Community College of Philadelphia. She was correcting care plans—what else? In frustration, she had written in bold letters across the top of the paper, **"Where is the person?"**

Because the acute hospital has become such a fast-paced, high-technology, short-stay, high-stimulus environment, it may very well have become a less effective teaching-learning environment for some aspects of nursing. Within this high-paced setting, it is often difficult for students to know individuals over time, to appreciate them as individuals with special histories, to hear their simple, yet powerful requests, "Excuse me nurse, I need to be home by 4 o'clock."

The nursing home, on the other hand, where nursing care is the critical variable in patient well-being, provides the opportunity to combine functional, cognitive, and physical assessment in planning care, to make nursing decisions over time and evaluate their effectiveness, to manage the impact of environment on a resident's condition, to work closely with nursing assistants, and to set goals and carry out nursing interventions that maintain or at best rehabilitate, but do not necessarily restore or cure. In the nursing home, students are provided an opportunity to create therapeutic environments away from the tubes and machines of the acute-care system, to step back for a brief moment and refocus on the caring mission of nursing.

"When we started here, I thought this was such a waste of time, but now I know that we are not just looking at illness, that you have to look at the whole person. I never thought about that before." Joyce, a second-year student who had just completed the nursing home clinical experience, speaks to the process of her knowing. Her story is captured on the video *Time to Care*. Her words tell the story of the nursing home, a care-oriented environment that, by its very nature, helps students and faculty to rethink essential beliefs about nursing and nursing practice. For Joyce, helping a resident, Mrs. Weinberg, become oriented to her surroundings became a mission. She cared about her and would somehow make her life better. Joyce lived the experience with Mrs. Weinberg over weeks and, in the process, she had time for reflection, for evaluation, for discouragement, and for trying again. As a teacher, I had time for support and encouragement, for stepping back and letting Joyce make her own choices about calendars and red tape along the hallway pointing the way to Mrs. Weinberg's room, and then for helping her find meaning in the outcome. In the end, Joyce discovered what was essential for Mrs. Weinberg—to be known as an individual and cared for in a familiar environment, to maintain her usual routine, to reach the end of the hall and ask a familiar but nameless face, "Excuse me nurse, is this the way to my room?" For Joyce, the belief that nursing care is directed toward the whole person, not just toward illness, became a meaningful concept, not just one she had verbalized in the classroom. Her ideas about nursing and nursing practice were transformed. Curriculum lives when it takes place in the context of reality.

In a classroom, weeks after our clinical experience in the nursing home, Joyce said to me, "You know Elaine, I've been thinking about Mrs. Weinberg and about our experiences in the nursing home and you know, life means so much more than just a heartbeat." Joyce came to know nursing home residents as individuals with special histories and unique needs. She learned to plan and implement nursing care directed toward promotion of optimal functional ability, maintenance of a familiar and safe environment, and pursuit of rehabilitation potential despite the presence of functional and cognitive impairment and chronic illness. Joyce experienced the sense of competence that comes from assisting older frail adults to improve and maintain their quality of life, without regard for their cure potential. The nursing home provided her with a rich environment to focus on these competencies, and these are the competencies that are essential if we are to be effective caregivers for older adults in any setting.

For faculty in project schools, supporting students in generalizing from the nursing home to other settings has become a major curriculum focus. If we are to help students begin to humanize the technological environments of the modern health care system, if we are to help students to see older adults differently and to see potential for growth and healing, then we must assist them to transfer learning from the care-focused environment of the nursing home to the acute-care setting and to recognize the value of maintenance, rehabilitation, and quality of life issues in both settings. And we know it can happen.

Susan, another second-year nursing student also featured in the video *Time to Care*, greeted me excitedly at graduation last May. She said,

> *You'll be so proud of me. Two weeks ago, when I arrived on the medical-surgical unit, I was told that my patient, Mr. Rogers, would need to go to a nursing home because he was unable to learn how to empty his supra-pubic catheter. The nurse had tried to teach him proper drainage techniques, but she said he just became confused and tearful. Since I knew Mr. Rogers had lived alone in an apartment before hospitalization and planned to return there to be with his friends, I decided to do a more thorough cognitive assessment. I met with him and we talked. I administered a standardized mental status examination slowly over the course of the evening and found he had excellent recall and was able to concentrate on activities. He was fully oriented. During that evening and the next, Mr. Rogers and I practiced emptying the bag over and over again. I kept telling him how much confidence I had in him and how well he was doing. When I charted at the end of the night, I made sure to describe his progress. When I came back the next time, I learned that he had been discharged to his home with referral to the community health nurse. I felt terrific. I look at older adults differently now. I don't accept*

statements about what they can't do. Being independent, living in an environment that is familiar and safe; well, that's so important.

Both Susan and Sarah's story illustrate that by understanding and knowing the older adult as an individual with special needs, we can create caring environments in any setting. Their stories, and your stories, must compel nurse educators to shift from a totally acute-care, hospital-based curriculum to caring environments like the nursing home. As we send our students out into the modern care system where older adults are the major recipients of nursing care, we owe them the opportunity and the knowledge base to respond to older adults as individuals and to meet their simple requests, requests that are not dramatic or even numerous. Olin asked every person who entered his room the same question: "Will I be home by 4:00?" Yet no one listened. Why? Because his one request, his one need, did not fit within the fast-paced, high-tech environment of the hospital. His need did not fit the cure-oriented focus of his caregivers. Olin wasn't asking for the cure for cancer; he wanted independence. He begged for the ability to function optimally in his own familiar environment and he asked only to be seen as an individual with continuity, who seeks quality to his living. These are the practice patterns that must drive nursing practice in the future.

On the other hand, none of us involved in the Community College–Nursing Home Partnership Project is advocating a curriculum where competence in high-tech care is not highly valued. We must educate nurses who understand the acute-care environment, who are competent practitioners, who can safely manipulate the tubes, the lines, and the equipment of the high-tech, acute-care system. But we shortchange our students, and our clients, if we do not recognize and teach the practice patterns so vividly played out in settings like the nursing home. We must shift our nursing practice paradigm or we will lose the person.

I believe this firmly. My father died last summer, in that hospital bed next to Olin. He spent his last days in the hospital, filled with cancer. On one of those days, as I entered his room, I heard him say weakly, "Excuse me nurse, I know I'm only on liquids but did I ever tell you that every morning, for as long as I can remember, I ate shredded wheat. Any chance I could have some now?" The "old" nurse in me heard only the absurdity of shredded wheat and a bowel obstruction. The transformed nurse in me, the one that has been changed by my experiences with the Community College–Nursing Home Partnership, and, more specifically, by understanding the essential practice patterns of the nursing home, that nurse listened differently. That nurse wished that just one of my father's caregivers had recognized the personal meaning in that simple request for shredded wheat. I've often thought of that moment with my father and about Olin and Anna. Joyce is right you know. Life means so much more than just a heartbeat. It means being home by 4:00; it means being recognized as an individual with worth, who knows a great deal about long rivers; and on a sunny June day, as life was slowly ebbing away, it meant shredded wheat.

5

Relationships in Clinical Teaching: The Faculty Role Revisited

Verle Waters

In 1986, the National League for Nursing issued a call for revolution in education. This curriculum revolution, like most interesting ideas, has given new meaning to a number of words and phrases, reflecting changes the revolution hoped to accomplish. *Behavioral objectives,* for example, once exalted as art, have been found guilty of tyranny. It amused me to hear about an author who submitted a proposal for a presentation at one of the nurse educator conferences, and true to the spirit of the revolution was unwilling to write behavioral objectives for the presentation. Still, continuing education requirements being what they are, there had to be objectives. Under duress, the author complied, but called them *subjectives.* A second phrase captures for me the essence of our topic: revolutionary writers enjoin us to let *"practice* inform *theory,"* rather than "apply theory to practice." Bevis (1991) puts it this way: "What the new nursing educational world order is about is a new relationship to reality, so that students and faculty are not isolated in education but are part and parcel of practice. With this relationship will come a reversal from 'What you learn in class today you will practice in clinical tomorrow' to 'What you experience in clinical today will be the focus for the class tomorrow.'"

Drawing upon the experiences of faculty and students in six community colleges in a clinical teaching and learning experience in nursing homes, I will describe in specific terms the change in faculty role which accompanies the switch from the teaching approach of "applying theory to practice" to one of "letting practice inform theory."

THE COMMUNITY COLLEGE–NURSING HOME PARTNERSHIP PROJECT

The Community College–Nursing Home Partnership project, initiated a few years before the outbreak of the curriculum revolution, had teachers in six colleges breaking new ground in devising a clinical experience in the nursing home for second-level students. (I might add that the faculty members who took on this new assignment were energetic and creative teachers, the type who look for new challenges.) By their accounts, when they began to develop a clinical in the nursing home, they started out using the same framework and approach they were accustomed to using when arranging clinical instruction in the hospital. Meeting with the head nurse or director of nursing in the nursing home, clinical objectives in hand or in mind, the faculty member would say, "We will be here tomorrow morning, my 10 students and I. I am here now to select patients for this assignment." "Residents," the nursing home nurse says. "Oh, yes, residents," the teacher says. "Very well. I want 10 patients—I mean residents—that are mentally able to relate to the students. I need four that have mobility problems, two with renal complications, and four with compromised cardiopulmonary function." About that time the nursing home staff member has a look on her face that seems to question the mental competence or at least the orientation of time and place of the faculty member.

The clinical instructors in our project soon abandoned that approach, and a somewhat trial-and-error period followed, aided by the opportunity to talk with peers in the other project schools. What emerged as the faculty members came to know the nursing home and design a quite different approach to the clinical teaching role bore serendipitous resemblance to the kind of teaching called for by the revolutionary writers and speakers. In this regard, Nelms (1991) defines curriculum as:

> *The educational journey, in an educational environment, in which biography of the person (the student) interacts with the history of the culture of nursing through the biography of another person (the faculty) to create meaning and release potential in the lives of all participants.*

If those first teachers in our project had had the option to quit the nursing home after the first trial, I have no doubt some of them would have quit, saying, "We can't meet our objectives in that setting." Such an option did not exist for them, however, because of the project commitment to devote at minimum three years of funding to a second-level clinical in the nursing home. As a result, there was time to think about what was going on. Tagliareni (1991) has observed about that period, "The nursing home environment was unfamiliar and faculty were outside of their comfort zone. The major issue, they began to realize, was not updated or expanded knowledge in gerontological nursing; rather it was confrontation of the long-established traditions of hospital-based learning and the search for value, opportunity, and comfort as a teacher in the nursing home." In a further observation about that period, Tagliareni said,

> *The faculty quickly discovered that the reactive model of clinical teaching, where the clinical instructor responds to available learning situations (dry IVs, a need for pain medication, crisis situations) does not work in the nursing home. Furthermore, faculty were accustomed to working in acute care where the instructor and students engage in parallel play—selecting a set of activities to carry out alongside the hospital nursing staff. In parallel play, the assigned client is often viewed by staff as being the responsibility of the faculty member and the nursing student. . . . Mutual care planning between student and staff is limited. Fortunately, parallel play is unsuited to the nursing home. Because nurses in nursing homes know the residents and their families intimately and because the residents value highly their relationships with familiar staff members, the faculty member must teach with, rather than next to, nursing staff.*

Since you are reading this and are interested, presumably, in clinical teaching, I suspect you have already discovered one of the bewildering facts about our nursing education literature. We write and talk (and think, by implication) much more about the selection, organization, and delivery of the didactic component than we do about the clinical component of nursing education. Isn't that surprising, since we are a practice discipline? I have two books in my library about clinical teaching: one, something of a classic, I suppose, by Infante, entitled *The Clinical Laboratory in Nursing Education,* and the other, published in 1985 by Reilly and Oermann from Wayne State University, is entitled *The Clinical Field: Its Use in Nursing Education* and presents a broader and more theoretical examination of the topic. Frankly, the most useful discussion of clinical education from my point of view is by two psychologists, Argyris and Schon.

Argyris and Schon (1974) believe that the clinical field has four central educational uses in professional education: (1) learning how to learn, (2) handling ambiguity, (3) thinking like professionals, and (4) developing personal causation.

Some years ago at Ohlone College we found the Argyris and Schon discussion on clinical learning helpful in developing a carefully structured placement for senior-level students with hospital staff-nurse preceptors. The experiences that thoughtful and talented teachers have had in taking on a clinical teaching role in the unfamiliar environment of the nursing home have sharpened once again the relevance of these four succinctly stated purposes of clinical education.

In the process of redefining the faculty role as clinical teachers in the nursing home, the faculty in the project made changes in the teacher-student relationship and in the teacher–nursing staff relationship. As a result, we found particular improvement in the learning outcomes identified as important by Argyris and Schon (1974). Students find more opportunities in nursing homes than in the acute-care hospital of today to take responsibility for their own learning, to plan and carry out nursing interventions in highly ambiguous situations, to contemplate and discuss the distinctive role of the nurse, and to experience the achievement of making a difference in the well-being of one or more residents.

As a result, power relationships between student and teacher changed. In some ways, this began with a dissatisfaction with the written care plan. Students wrote volumes—residents in nursing homes have multilayered and multicolored health problems—and yet the factor or problem most relevant to the day-to-day life of the resident might still be missed. As Tanner (1988) has observed, understanding the lived experiences of illness and frailty escapes the formalizations of the traditional nursing care plan approach.

Rather than asking students to create care plans each week on an individual basis, two practices emerged that changed student-faculty power relationships: students were invited to pick one resident as their primary focus, and to share care-planning thoughts and processes with the instructor. Again, quoting from Tagliareni's (1991) account of this process:

> *A series of questions emerged in our thinking: is it not time for us to begin the practice of collegiality with students? To share care planning, for example, rather than asking second-level students to prove to me*

each week that they are capable of rediscovering a plan of care? Why do students need to go in cold each week to assess clients, determine behavior outcomes, and generate nursing interventions? Is it any wonder that they run out of time to individualize, to find the person? We concluded that in the nursing home setting, students would be assigned the same group of residents for the entire experience. Each student shares at least one client with the instructor; together they conduct assessments, co-lead reminiscing activity groups, and brainstorm about creative approaches to care.

A second change in relationships was prompted by faculty dissatisfaction with the traditional care plan assignment, namely faculty actively promoting peer relationships among students. Students are organized into teams of three or four students per team and assigned a group of residents as a team. The student group writes care plans together for each of the residents and critiques these in post-conference. Students ask each other: could I provide individualized care for this resident after reading this care plan? How can phrases like "be consistent" or "establish trust" be made meaningful and specific for each resident?

Completing this triad that Bevis (1991) calls the "tripartite alliance" in education, a different set of relationships emerged between faculty and nursing home staff, and between students and nursing home staff.

This change began with an awakening to a new attitude toward the nursing home nurse. Nursing homes have been at the bottom of the nursing totem pole, afforded status well below that afforded the intensive-care nurse, for example. As we know, until quite recently, nursing education, along with all other health professions, has virtually ignored the nursing home and the nurses who work there.

Respect for the nurses and other staff who work in nursing homes grew, and with a more enlightened and expanded view of them as professionals and caregivers, faculty initiated learning activity structures that drew staff actively into the equation, allowing them to become full partners in the learning enterprise and socializing students in the development and maintenance of relationships with fellow workers that are quite different from those in the acute-care clinical.

Clinical practice is more than the opportunity to put theory learned in the classroom into practice. Benner (1983) notes that "theory offers what can be made explicit and formalized, but clinical practice is always more complex and presents many more realities than can be captured by theory alone." The faculty in the Community College–Nursing Home Partnership have found the nursing home an extraordinary and valuable clinical environment for successful teaching of those complexities and realities.

REFERENCES

Argyris, C., & Schon, D. (1974). *Theory in practice: Increasing professional effectiveness.* San Francisco: Jossey-Bass.

Benner, P. (1983). *From novice to expert.* Menlo Park, CA: Addison-Wesley. p. 36.

Bevis, E. O. (1991). *Building new educational relationships: The future is now.* SREB Annual Meeting, October, 1991.

Infante, M. S. (1975). *The Clinical Laboratory in Nursing Education.* New York: John Wiley & Sons.

Nelms, T. P. (1991, January). Has the curriculum revolution revolutionized the definition of curriculum? *Journal of Nursing Education, 30,* 1.

Reilly, D. E., & Oermann, M. H. (1985). *The clinical field: Its use in nursing education.* Norwalk, CT: Appleton-Century-Crofts.

Tagliareni, E. (1991). What and how of student learning activities. In V. Waters (Ed.), *Teaching gerontology.* New York: National League for Nursing.

Tanner, C. (1988). Curriculum revolution: The practice mandate. *Nursing and Health Care, 9,* 427–430.

6

Gerontologic Nursing Competency Development: Associate Degree in Nursing & Bachelor of Science in Nursing: History—Commonalities—Differences

Susan Sherman and Mary Burke

One ship sails east an another sails west
With the self-same wind that blows
Tis the set of the sails and not the gales
That determines the way they go.
Like the winds of the sea are the winds of fate
As we journey along through life.
Tis the set of the soul that determines the goal
And not the calm or the strife.

Ella Wheeler Wilcox

In the late 1980s, the multiple concerns of nurse educators regarding the health care needs of the aging population, the issues of relevant curricula, and the need for realistic expectations of graduates prompted the initiation of two parallel but independent competency development activities. The impetus for these endeavors emerged from previous and ongoing demonstration projects—the Community College–Nursing Home Partnership, funded by the W.K. Kellogg Foundation, the Teaching

Nursing Home Project funded by the Robert Wood Johnson Foundation, and the Gerontologic Nursing Education Continuing Care Project, funded by the Division of Nursing, United States Public Health Service, Department of Health and Human Services. These three projects challenged faculty to use nursing homes as clinical settings for student learning. Experiences of project faculty resulted in a systematic identification of the knowledge, skills, and values necessary for the practice of gerontologic nursing. As the importance of systematic curriculum revision became evident to both groups of faculty, sponsorship of independent competency development activities occurred.

Both associate degree (ADN) and baccalaureate degree (BSN) competency activities, using a consensus-building process, developed competency statements without recognition, input, or dialogue with each other. It is remarkable that an analysis of the two sets of statements completed by the authors reveal a shared vision of improved care for the elderly and a mutual concern for the need to prepare effective caregivers for older adults. For too long nursing educators from ADN and BSN programs have worked parallel to and isolated from each other in their preparation of graduates to address the health care needs of various populations. This dual approach has contributed to the fragmentation of nursing education and has weakened the image of nursing.

In a practice world where communication among health care providers is essential, where team approaches to problem solving are critical, and where building on mutual strengths is fundamental, nursing can no longer ignore the imperative to foster collaboration among its educators and its practitioners. Dialogue within nursing is necessary if the social mandate to provide responsible health care to older Americans is to be fully realized. Mutual vision emerges through dialogue that embodies mutual understanding and mutual respect.

It is in this spirit of collaboration that faculty from Georgetown University School of Nursing and faculty from the Community College–Nursing Home Partnership (CC–NHP) began their journey into the analysis of two sets of gerontologic competencies for nursing graduates.

THE COMMUNITY COLLEGE–NURSING HOME PARTNERSHIP

From 1986 to 1990, a six-college project funded by the W.K. Kellogg Foundation, titled The Community College–Nursing Home Partnership: Improving Care Through Education, addressed two seminal objectives: (1) developing nursing potential in nursing homes through inservice education for staff and (2) redirecting associate degree nursing to encompass preparation for nursing roles in long-term care as well as acute care.

Competency Development

Associated with the ADN gerontologic competency development was a provision for a two-day meeting of 12 registered nurses from nursing homes, two from each of the national project school sites. Employing a process known as DACUM (an acronym for *Developing A Curriculum*), the nurses were asked to systematically identify the competencies for registered nurse practice in the nursing home setting. Their work resulted in a list of over 300 competencies within 18 categories describing the clinical skills, knowledge, and behaviors needed for safe and effective practice in the nursing home. Further analysis of the competencies revealed that while many were universal to nursing practice in any setting, some were unique to both the nursing home setting and to the care of frail elderly clients with multiple chronic health problems. Project faculty identified 25 specific competencies as essential learning outcomes appropriate for associate degree nursing graduates to master and best taught in a nursing home environment. These competencies have formed the core curriculum outcomes for ADN nursing home clinical experiences and have served as guidelines for nursing home staff development. The competency language, concise and pragmatic, is that of nurses working in nursing homes.

Those competency statements "best taught" within the core curriculum are reflected in the 1990 NLN–CADP (National League for Nursing–Council of Associate Degree Programs) statement, *Educational Outcomes of Associate Degree Nursing Programs: Roles and Competencies*.

A dissemination phase of the Community College–Nursing Home Partnership has also included collaborative activities with regulatory and accrediting bodies to support increased curricular attention to gerontological nursing. A significant relationship was developed between the dissemination project and the concurrent effort to revise and update the 1978 NLN–CADP "Competencies of the Associate Degree Nurse on Entry into Practice."

Community College–Nursing Home Partnership: National Influence on ADN Curricula

"Best taught" competencies were studied, along with other contemporary evidence, as the NLN committee pursued the broadest possible understanding of current and future practice patterns of associate degree nurses. The resulting document, *Education Outcomes of Associate Degree Nursing Programs: Roles and Competencies* (1990), addresses the nursing needs of an aging population in emphasizing knowledge and skills required to serve the elderly population, to manage client care resources, to think critically, and to embrace values and practice ethically. These NLN–CADP competencies specifically address the preparation of registered nurses to provide direct care to clients across the life span, with an emphasis on adults. Three roles are identified as basic to associate degree nursing practice: provider of care, manager of care, and member within the discipline of nursing. Within each role, concern for the older client is emphasized, as is the need for the development of practice patterns unique to both acute and long-term care settings. Drawing attention to the distinctive relationship between practice pattern and setting makes the document particularly useful for program development and graduate assessment.

For example, within the provider of care role, practice is characterized by:

> *critical thinking, clinical competence, accountability, and a commitment to the value of care. This practice applies to clients across the life span with emphasis on adults who have health needs and require assistance to maintain or restore their optimum states of health or support to die with dignity. Because the aged comprise an increasing proportion of nursing clients, the nurse with an associate degree is prepared to address the acute and chronic health needs of this population.* (Education Outcomes of Associate Degree Nursing Programs: Roles and Competencies, 1990, p. 3).

The client population of the associate degree nursing graduate is defined as individuals under care, each possessing relationships with family, group, and community. Decision making is guided by the nursing process; collaboration is a practice methodology. Graduates are prepared for nursing practice in both acute and long-term care settings where policies and procedures are specified and guidance is available.

Some of the competency statements in the NLN–CADP document evolved specifically from the experience of the CC–NHP faculty as teachers in the nursing home. These include:

- Participates with the client, family, significant others, and members of the health care team to establish client-centered goals directed toward promoting and restoring the client's optimum state of health, preventing illness, and providing rehabilitation.
- Supports clients' right to make decisions regarding care.
- Promotes an environment conducive to maintenance or restoration of the client's ability to carry out activities of daily living.
- Promotes the rehabilitation potential of the client.
- Provides for continuity of care in the management of chronic health care needs.
- Demonstrates caring behavior in providing nursing care.

Within the manager of care role, practice is characterized by "collaboration, organization, delegation, accountability, advocacy, and respect for other health care workers." This statement points out that delegating aspects of care to licensed and unlicensed personnel commensurate with their educational backgrounds and experience is a component of accountability. Again, the practice setting is defined as the acute or long-term care setting where policies and procedures are specified and where guidance is available.

Manager of care competencies that evolved specifically from faculty experience in the nursing home include:

- Assists other nursing personnel to develop skills in providing nursing care.
- Practices in a cost-effective manner.
- Manages an environment that promotes clients' self-esteem, dignity, safety, and comfort.
- Promotes effective team relationships.
- Is accountable for performance of nursing activities delegated to other workers.
- Participates in evaluation of the client care delivery system.

Finally, within the role, practice is characterized by "a commitment to professional growth, continuous learning, and self-development . . .

within the ethical and legal framework of nursing and is responsible for ensuring high standards of nursing practice" (*Education Outcomes of Associate Degree Nursing Programs: Roles and Competencies*, 1990, p. 10).

Statements of competencies that also reflect increased emphasis on ethical issues and role modeling include:

- Values nursing as a career and values own practice.
- Recognizes and reports ethical dilemmas encountered in practice.
- Constructs a course of action when confronted with ethical dilemmas in practice.
- Serves as a role model to members of the nursing team.
- Recognizes the importance of nursing research in advancing nursing practice.
- Participates in research conducted at the employing institution.

Within the shift in curricular emphasis for associate degree nursing education as represented in the 1990 NLN–CADP competency document, certain values are emphasized over others, including: the practice role in long-term care; a de-emphasis of the specialty areas of maternal, child, and mental health nursing; a reflection of recent job analyses (Kane et al., 1986); and a response to recent national demographic shifts within the job market. Further, this new emphasis on job analyses and demography is necessary to prepare practitioners for a world where they will spend approximately 75 percent of their work lives caring for clients over the age of 65.

Because the four "best taught" gerontologic competency categories (Perform a Resident Assessment, Practice Rehabilitation Nursing Skills, Manage the Living Environment, and Exhibit Management Skills) comprise current expectations for student learning, faculty have had to re-examine their teaching methods. Learning experiences developed within these categories support student understanding of the meaning of valuing and maintaining individualization of care, the caring mission of nursing, understanding clients differently, recognizing and valuing rehabilitation potential and optimum functioning, understanding quality of life, and developing collaborative relationships with staff. In this regard, faculty have been challenged to shed practice patterns that work well in acute care but not in long-term care settings and to share with students an understanding of nursing education as a mentoring, coaching, and supportive process of learning.

DEVELOPMENT OF THE BACCALAUREATE COMPETENCIES

In the 1980s, the Georgetown University School of Nursing was the recipient of two major gerontologic funding initiatives, one private and the other government (the Robert Wood Johnson Teaching Nursing Home Project and the Gerontologic Nursing Education Continuing Care Project). The projects allowed for a cadre of gerontologic nurse educators to work together at one school at one point in time. At Georgetown, our past involvement with the Robert Wood Johnson Teaching Nursing Home Project became the common ground for faculty to pursue their research. These faculty, along with other like-minded colleagues, also became members of the new project, the Gerontologic Nursing Education Continuing Care Project, funded by the Division of Nursing, U.S. Public Health Service, Department of Health and Human Services.

This experience allowed the faculty to address the critical and timely issue of what gerontologic knowledge and skills are requisite for the beginning baccalaureate nursing graduate. Shared faculty goals led to the planning, initiation, and implementation of the National Invitational Gerontologic Consensus Conference to Identify Gerontologic Nursing Competencies for Baccalaureate Graduates. With corporate funding and university support for the conference, 18 nursing leaders of gerontologic education, practice, and administration were brought to Georgetown for an intensive two-day consensus workshop.

Dr. Thelma Wells opened the conference with a keynote address on the history of competency development in gerontologic nursing education. She urged participants not only to develop competencies but also to address the appropriate dissemination of the results of the conference. Dr. Mary Stull, a consultant for competency development, led the conference workshop within the context of a modified nominal group process to facilitate competency development. The participants, divided into three groups with an equal mix of educators, practitioners, and administrators, chose the nursing process as the organizing factor to develop beginning competency statements.

The three groups of experts identified the knowledge essential for gerontologic nursing and the nurse caring attributes desired for older adults. By the end of the conference, the invited participants had agreed to continue volunteering their time and effort to complete the necessary competency validation. Two drafts were sent for validation: the first for confirmation of content and intent and the second for leveling between baccalaureate and master's (gerontologic nursing specialization) preparation.

Included in the drafts are competencies that are pertinent to and warrant specific emphasis for the care of older adults. These competencies, however, are not inclusive of all competencies that are identified in most baccalaureate curricula. Divided into two major headings (Professional Practice and Nursing Process), the competencies were published in 1992 by the National League for Nursing in *Gerontology in the Nursing Curriculum*.

THE COMMONALITIES

An analysis of the ADN and BSN competency statements reveal similarities in knowledge base, skills, and values needed by nurses to be safe, competent caregivers of frail older adults with chronic health problems. These commonalities include practice patterns grounded in a problem-solving approach, the nursing process, and an understanding of rehabilitation principles that maintain and support a restorative care focus. Special emphasis is placed on valuing and understanding the multiple environments where the frail elderly reside and receive care, as well as a rethinking of care models that support individualized care within these environments. Furthermore, the integration of management roles into all levels of practice patterns and a respect for legal and ethical aspects essential for practice, including honesty, confidentiality, clients' rights for decision making, informed consent, and autonomy, were important elements in both competency statements.

THE DIFFERENCES

Differences, however, do exist in the competencies and outcome statements, including differences in setting, definition of client population, and resources utilized by graduates. Whereas the setting for practice of the ADN graduate is defined as the acute and long-term care environments with policies and procedures specified and guidance available, the setting for practice of the BSN graduate is defined more broadly as any interface of the nurse and the older person, their significant others, and the community.

Client populations targeted for the ADN graduate are primarily individual residents within the context of their significant group. For BSN graduates, the target group is somewhat larger and includes individuals, significant others, groups, and community. Perhaps the most obvious differences in practice patterns of BSN and ADN graduates involves BSN participation in interdisciplinary team activities. Although the ADN graduate can make valuable contributions to a resident's data base and to interdisciplinary team planning, the knowledge base of the BSN graduate incorporates additionally important aspects: practice guided by nursing theory and based on research findings, management of resources, evaluation of the complexity of client needs in community settings, and development of health promotion strategies for individuals and communities. Finally, BSN competencies speak to an involvement in clinical research and an understanding of the regulatory process as viable elements in the planning of care.

Behaviors of different graduates from different types of educational preparation should be carefully examined to support the strengths each bring to the setting and to the practice of nursing care of the frail older adult.

CONCLUSION

Consultation and collaboration between nursing educators of associate degree and baccalaureate programs does not have an enlightened history. Unfortunately, the norm has been to maintain distance and emphasize differences rather than commonalities between the two types of programs. Rather than becoming embroiled in the educational issues that continue to divide the profession, we recognized the greater need to focus on the elderly, frail person as a recipient of nursing care. It is nursing care to elderly, frail clients that must be improved by the enhanced education of practitioners from all levels of nursing, students and staff alike.

In spite of differences, the common bond of mutual respect and the recognition of the importance of dialogue led the participants of both competency development conferences to an affiliation with the National League for Nursing for the joint sponsorship of the gerontologic conference. Every gerontologic nurse, whether ADN or BSN graduate, shares a similar vision: health care for elderly Americans should be affordable, and should foster autonomy, promote health, provide excellent illness care, and support a death with dignity. This is the vision of committed nurses. Unity of purpose and support of health care reform will bring this vision to reality. For this and other reasons, we will continue our efforts toward continued collaboration and consultation within nursing education and with nursing service.

REFERENCES

Council of Associate Degree Programs (1992). *Educational outcomes of associate degree programs: Roles and competencies.* New York: National League for Nursing.

Kane, M., Kingsbury, C., Colton D., & Estes, C. (1986). *A study of nursing practice and role delineation and job analyses of entry-level performance of registered nurses.* Chicago: National Council of State Boards of Nursing, Inc.

Gerontology in the Nursing Curriculum (1992). New York: National League for Nursing.

Tagliareni, E., Sherman, S., Waters, V., & Mengel, A. (1991, May). Participatory clinical education: Reconceptualizing the clinical learning environment. *Nursing and Health Care, 12*:5.

7

Facilitating Student Learning: Effective Teaching Strategies for Baccalaureate Education

Norma R. Small

Gerontological nursing education, and the dearth thereof, has become a focus of concern among employers, consumers, students, and educators. The knowledge and skills of the baccalaureate-prepared nurse are changing with the changing demographics of the client population. Increasingly, this client population is older, is better educated about health care, has multiple chronic diseases, and is being treated with more sophisticated medical technology. Knowledge learned about the 35-year-old cannot be applied to the over-85-year-old, the fastest growing segment of the population and the age group consuming the largest portion of health care dollars.

Nursing, as well as other health care professions, has been slow to recognize the different approaches to health care delivery necessitated by the aging of the population. Schools of nursing have attempted to integrate gerontological nursing into the curriculum with varying, usually discouraging, amounts of success. The lack of general acceptance of a gerontological focus in the curriculum, as exists currently with pediatrics, has been attributed to several factors: (1) knowledge unique to gerontologic nursing is not tested on the NCLEX in proportion to the client population, (2) there is no consensus as to what basic knowledge and skills should be taught, and (3) most faculty members have not had formal preparation in gerontological nursing and are not comfortable teaching didactic or clinical gerontological nursing.

PROBLEMS IN TEACHING GERONTOLOGICAL NURSING

The first factor, inclusion on the NCLEX, can only be accomplished when there is consensus on the basic knowledge unique to gerontologic nursing necessary for entry into nursing practice. The second factor, determining gerontological knowledge, skills, and competencies to be taught at the baccalaureate level requires consensus by educators. This was accomplished at the National Invitational Consensus Conference to Identify Gerontologic Nursing Competencies for Baccalaureate Graduates held at Georgetown University in 1990 (Small, Burke, & Maddox, 1991). The third factor, faculty preparation in gerontological nursing, requires a change of faculty attitudes about gerontological nursing and a commitment to attend faculty development programs on gerontological nursing teaching strategies.

In this chapter, I will discuss some teaching strategies to integrate gerontological nursing concepts into a baccalaureate curriculum. Immediate goals of these gerontological nursing teaching strategies include: (1) promoting a positive attitude toward older persons and the care of older persons; (2) creating a positive learning environment appropriate to student learning needs, style, and abilities; (3) motivating students to acquire the necessary knowledge and skills in gerontological nursing for beginning baccalaureate graduates; and (4) integrating gerontological nursing concepts in all teaching-learning opportunities. In order to determine what teaching strategies can be used in baccalaureate nursing education, the academic setting, the curriculum, the students, and the faculty must be considered.

Academic setting involves the position of the nursing program within the parent institution and the control the nursing program retains in regard to number of credits and the required core curriculum offered. Philosophy of baccalaureate education and the value placed on professional versus liberal arts education also influence the time available and the resources allocated. The geographical location of the institution, of course, will dictate the clinical practice opportunities available.

Curriculum is the responsibility of the faculty and reflects faculty values and philosophy of nursing education. The new National League for Nursing accreditation criteria allows for greater creativity and uniqueness in a curriculum within five basic outcome parameters, one being the pass rate on the NCLEX. The theoretical framework and terminal objectives offered will exert substantial influence on the degree to which gerontological concepts are integrated into the full curriculum. The organizational framework of the curriculum, such as life cycle, continuum of care, and integrated versus medical model, will also determine where and how gerontology will be taught. The specificity of course objectives and the degree of academic freedom instructors have in meeting these objectives will determine the degree to which gerontology is integrated into the full curriculum. Instructors usually teach content that is most familiar to them. With time constraints and broad objectives that state "across the life span," the latter third of the life span is frequently overlooked or dealt with superficially unless a commitment to gerontologic nursing exists within the nursing program as a whole.

Student characteristics such as maturity, past experiences, and motivation are important factors to be considered in choosing teaching strategies. Some students come to the learning environment highly motivated to care for older persons based on prior, positive experiences with older family members and neighbors. Other students come with negative attitudes toward their own aging and older persons learned from the media and societal values. They may also have an unrealistic view of nursing as "high-tech" medicine instead of the "high-touch" caring focus appropriate to gerontological nursing.

Faculty members and their educational preparation, clinical expertise, and attitudes toward aging form the last major factor in nursing education that must be considered. Most faculty members did not have specific gerontological nursing content in their basic preparation and especially not in their advanced preparation in a clinical specialty, unless that was gerontological nursing. Most faculty members feel uncomfortable teaching clinical content in an area other than that in which they have expertise. To complicate the matter, clients assigned to students to meet specific learning objectives may be older persons. The student's instructor may not have had the knowledge or skills necessary to teach the student the unique aspects of how older persons experience illness, how to respond to the multidisciplinary management necessary in such care, or how to adapt nursing interventions to meet the unique needs of an aging client. In fact, the reluctance to recognize the unique nursing needs and learning opportunities presented by older persons may reflect societal attitudes toward aging as well as faculty members' denial of the aging process that they or their parents are experiencing. As such, faculty members' philosophies of teaching and knowledge of how students learn are important components of their ability to teach gerontological nursing. Do faculty teach content over which they have control or do they take risks by teaching students how to learn via the spirit of inquiry?

GOALS OF GERONTOLOGICAL TEACHING STRATEGIES

The first goal of a teaching strategy is to promote a positive attitude toward and a caring for older persons. In general, attitudes are affective tendencies based on learned beliefs that are used to evaluate an object and to predispose an individual to respond in a certain way. Beliefs about an object are learned from family, society, and the media. In this case, beliefs about older persons can result in positive (e.g., they are active and independent) or negative (e.g., they are stubborn and frail) attitudes. While attitudes are not the sole predictor of behavior, they do predispose a person to respond in a certain way. However, attitudes change whenever a person is exposed to new, more compelling information or experiences that conflict with the current attitude.

Clearly, faculty and clinical agency staff members' attitudes exert great influence over student attitudes and learning. As a result, it is important to assess attitudes toward aging and older persons. If attitudes toward older persons are negative, faculty and staff development workshops should be planned to "desensitize" the faculty and staff members' fear of their own aging. Faculty and staff members must also be provided sufficient "compelling" new knowledge and skills, based on current research and positive experiences with well older persons, to change prevailing, negative attitudes.

Learning situations must be designed and organized to change negative attitudes to positive attitudes. In this regard, students must have a positive presentation of gerontological nursing both in the classroom and in clinical practice. Gerontological content must also be based on the most current research available. Student clinical experiences should begin with well older persons who are models of coping and surviving in the face of multiple life changes. Students should not be placed in a clinical situation until they have the didactic knowledge and skills to deal with the other sorts of clients they will encounter, such as a very frail and demented older person in a nursing home. An initial clinical experience with a frail, demented, or chronically ill older person may, in fact, work against the dissemination of appropriate clinical content, reinforcing the student's stereotypical attitudes about older persons and devaluing the complexity of the clinical decision making required in the nursing management of such clients.

The second goal of a teaching strategy is to create a learning environment appropriate to the student's learning needs, style, and abilities. An appropriate learning environment for gerontological nursing begins with a positive attitude toward the care of older persons by the instructor, whether in the classroom, clinical area, or individual conference. Because of the large amount of content that must be covered in the time constraints of a curriculum, each learning activity must meet several objectives. While teaching the nursing management of a particular disease process, for example, the instructor could use case examples to compare and contrast the management of an adult, an older adult with normal aging changes, and an older adult with a concomitant chronic disease. The number of case examples using an older person should be in the same proportion as the incidence of the disease or health problem in the older adult population compared with younger age groups. Faculty members with expertise in gerontological nursing can serve as resources in developing case presentations and integration strategies. Older persons from the community or organizations such as the American Association of Retired Persons (AARP) can also serve as excellent resources and as guest speakers.

Experiential learning through interactions with older persons via role and game playing are effective means of reinforcing concepts. More mature and creative students can develop new games or adapt existing games (e.g., Trivial Pursuit or Jeopardy) to teach concepts about aging. Students can be challenged to be creative in meeting objectives through contracting for individualized projects. A long-term relationship with an older person to learn individual and family coping responses to the many challenges of aging is usually quite beneficial, especially for students who have not experienced a close relationship with grandparents or other older persons.

Clinical experiences should be designed to progress from simple to complex clinical decision making. For the older person, this developmental span includes the student assuming the role of health educator for the independent older person living in the community to the student managing the complex care interventions for the dependent older person in an acute or long-term care situation. Clients exhibiting this continuum of complexity can be found in community sites, such as churches and synagogues, senior centers, congregate housing, life care communities, long-term care agencies, and acute-care institutions. Agencies themselves are usually eager to have students stimulating their staff and clients with their creative ideas. Although students with a well-planned gerontological nursing experience do not necessarily choose gerontology as their specialty upon graduation, most of them learn to appreciate the need for specialists in this complex and growing area of health care.

The third goal of a teaching strategy is to motivate students to acquire the necessary knowledge and skills in gerontological nursing for beginning practice as a generalist. To implement this strategy, desired knowledge and skills must be identified. Conferences, the dissemination of conference papers, and other publications aid in this process. In the present conference, our goal was to identify minimum outcome criteria acceptable to gerontological nursing educators, practitioners, and administrators. Flexibility in the educational process to achieve such competencies is desirable. Motivating students to value the knowledge of such competencies requires enthusiasm and creativity among all faculty members whether or not they have gerontological nursing expertise. Integration of these competencies into the licensure examination (NCLEX) would be a further motivator for both faculty to teach gerontological nursing concepts and for students to learn them. This goal is yet to be achieved.

The fourth goal of a teaching strategy is to integrate gerontological nursing concepts into all teaching-learning opportunities. It is estimated that from 60 to 80 percent of acute-care hospital bed days are occupied by persons over age 65, and most of long-term care expenditures are for persons over age 65. Since gerontological nursing clients are integrated in all components of the health care continuum, it is a practical and sound teaching principle to integrate the care of older persons in all courses. Even the valuable role of grandparenting can be taught in maternal-child health courses. Unfortunately, psychiatric-mental health courses often overlook the needs of older persons, thereby contributing to their underrepresentation in the population of clients receiving mental health services despite the increased need of older persons for such services.

Foundational courses frequently taught by non-nursing faculty are important courses in which to integrate aging concepts. Anatomy and physiology courses should include content specific to normal changes of aging and the genetic influences at work in the aging process. Human growth and development courses should devote a proportionate amount of time to the last third of the life span. Pathophysiology courses should include the different presentations of diseases and symptoms with increasing age. The 85-year-old, for example, does not respond to a heart attack in the same way as the 45-year-old who is too much used as the "text book picture" even though heart disease incidence increases with age. Pharmacology is also a discipline that is just beginning to identify the aging changes in response to drugs by including older persons in drug trials.

Traditional clinical settings for teaching gerontological nursing, such as nursing homes, should be considered for teaching many acute-care skills in a nonthreatening environment. Nursing homes offer many experiences with medication administration, intravenous fluids, tube feedings, respirators, multiple system failure management, pre- and postoperative care, and in making complex decisions with the individual and family. Faculty members with gerontological nursing expertise must be assertive and enthusiastic when they approach other faculty about integrating gerontological nursing concepts into their courses and be readily available for consultation in the planning and implementation of this integration.

Effective learning of gerontological nursing concepts requires a clear statement of minimal expectations (competencies), faculty committed in all courses to teaching gerontology based on the latest research and packaged in a creative way, and faculty with gerontological nursing expertise to serve as enthusiastic and creative consultants. Creative strategies in integrating gerontological nursing into the already crowded curriculum need to be developed and disseminated. Baccalaureate nursing curricula must reflect the nursing care needs of society and the changing needs of the health care system.

8

*About Anger and Power**

Patricia Moccia

This chapter is about *anger* and *power* and the relationship between the two. It is also about the risks involved in nurses feeling and expressing their anger and power.

In this context, I will discuss gerontological nursing and the issues and opportunities in the field. I will explore some ideas of nursing's visions for an alternative health care system, and visions of alternative ways for us to "be" with each other—alternative ways to interact as citizens of our communities, to work together as professional colleagues, and to collaborate with our patients in the interest of health and healing.

Because I was so pleased with your invitation to talk with you and hear your ideas and visions about long-term care, I will also talk about inspiring a vision for long-term care and, just as importantly, how to substantiate such a vision. But I must do so in the context I have chosen, by discussing anger and power.

OUR CURRENT REALITIES: THE FRAME OF REFERENCE FOR OUR DISCUSSIONS

Why change the frame of reference? Why anger and power? Because Simone de Beavoir has told us that: "Representation of the world, like

---

* An abbreviated version of this paper and sections of it have been published previously in *Humanistic Psychology* and the *Journal of Nursing Education*.

the world itself, is the work of men; they describe it from their own point of view, which they confuse with the absolute truth."

And in their representation of the world, in the truth that they represent as the absolute truth, men have left little room for any public discussion of anger and power and clearly no room at all for women discussing such phenomena.

Over the centuries, the works of men have clearly been realities of dualities and polarities. These realities are built on a great and precarious divide, a gaping chasm, with theory divorced from practice, reason from passion, objective experiences from subjective experiences. In such realities the public sector was and is neatly delineated from the private sector with behaviors appropriate and inappropriate for each sector clearly identified and reinforced.

For an interlocking set of reasons, these constructed realities have become the status quo and the dominant forces present themselves as the only true reality. This reality, however monumental it may seem, is precarious and easily challenged, for example, by any crossover between public and private behaviors, when men are homemakers or nurses, when women are construction workers or run for political office. The status quo is also challenged at a deep and primal level when any feelings are expressed in a public forum such as this, outside the private sector to which feelings are normally relegated and where feelings more comfortably reside.

When those feelings are anger and power, and especially when the people expressing anger and power are women, then the act becomes something more than a challenge. Discussing anger and power, sharing our experiences about both, contributes to the deconstruction and rebuilding of the status quo. When discussing anger and power as nurses and healers and women, I also ask you to consider whether such a discussion is a necessary precondition to creating the knowledge that is needed for health. In my view the answer is yes. Discussing anger and power is a necessary precondition to both the inspiration and articulation of our visions of long-term care in the twenty-first century.

I want to discuss long-term care in the context of anger and power for still other reasons. May Sarton, in her 1988 work *After The Stroke*, speaks about the joy experienced when a frame of reference is suddenly widened. Our frame of reference is suddenly widened when we read the works of the great writer and witness of the 1930s, Meridel Le Sueur. From the Midwest, originally Minnesota and then from the Bay area of California, Le Sueur is described as a woman "whose ardor, energy and sense of commitment are undiminished by age." Rediscovered in the 1970s and 1980s, Le

Sueur writes in a multilayered, multidimensional way as a deliberate alternative to the linear narratives that Le Sueur sees as a male style directed toward a target and a conclusion to be appropriated. Her view of the world—as a web of interrelated parts, organic, of a whole, nonlinear, a universe of process, growth, and an energy that ever renews itself—has, I think, relevance for our thinking about gerontology and long-term care in a different way and within a different frame of reference.

Yet how shall we convince our colleagues and our politicians that they should be concerned about issues of long-term care? Shall we play to their kindness? To their sense of responsibility? To their empathy and ethics? Yes, of course, we should do all these. But an even more significant change can be effected if we change their frame of reference. Let us lead them to the joy of experiencing not only their relationship of responsibility to the aged, not only their relationship of empathy, but most significantly their relationship of identity.

And by that term I do not only mean identity in the sense, however powerful it might be, that we all one day will be old, or solely in the sense that we are always preparing to be old; as M.F.K. Fisher writes in *Sister Age*, "The art of aging is learned subtly but firmly" (p. 5). Rather let us offer a frame of reference that develops from the worldview that we are a whole. In Gregory Bateson's words, we are connected through an ecology of the mind. In our private and public worlds, our identity with the aging is of the same stuff—a nonlinear, multidimensional experience of connection with aging in our society; specifically, the connection of being different. *From this connection, this diversity, will come our greatest strength, our visions, and their substance and actualization.*

Thus, the reason for discussing the subject at hand—anger and power—is to share the joy of a political act, the exciting experience of political work in the public sphere. That this is a joy previously denied to women, and especially to nurses, must not deter us, for it is a joy that is finally at hand.

ABOUT ANGER

To what kind of anger am I referring? About which feelings?

I am referring to the anger we feel as nurses when we read in both the popular media and the trade press of prevailing solutions to current health crises that avoid questions about the dominance of the biomedical paradigm or the continued dominance of organized medicine.

I am referring to the anger we feel as researchers, begging for a measly $50,000 or $100,000 to start our projects of health and healing, and being told the federal well is dry. Yet, just a year ago, billions of dollars were blown away as 85,000 tons of nonnuclear "conventional" bombs were dropped on Iraq and Kuwait, wreaking more devastation than "five Hiroshimas" in what a United Nations observation team called "near-apocalyptical results" (Klare, 1991, p. 738).

I am referring to the anger of women researchers and the anger of researchers concerned with women's health when we compare the $80 million in the last federal budget that was allocated to research on breast cancer in women compared with the $240 million spent on Tomahawk missiles, only one of the many varieties of weapons used in the Persian Gulf, the $250 million spent for only two days of air combat, the $500 million spent for one day of air and ground combat, and the $12.3 billion spent for non-combat costs between January and March 1991 (Center for Defense Information, 1991).

I am referring to the anger of clinicians working in agencies funded with Title X monies who find themselves compromised as professionals and threatened as citizens by a gag rule imposed by the reactionary and mean-spirited Bush administration and tightened by a Supreme Court whose presiding justices seem impoverished of experiences other than those provided by their own sheltered worlds.

I am referring to the anger we feel working in long-term care within the strangulating limits of governmental support to nursing homes that in 1990 amounted to $99 per capita.

I am referring to the anger that comes with the knowledge that 84 percent of Americans between the ages of 65 and 79 cannot afford the average cost of basic nursing home insurance and 73 percent can't afford the lowest price long-term care coverage.

I am referring to the anger that accompanies working families forced into impoverishment in order to receive federal monies for catastrophic long-term care.

I am referring to the anger of working with families with AIDS patients in long-term care no one else will care for—AIDS patients—our wonderful youth—the potential of our country suffering and dying as the government's research agenda into HIV infections seems, at times, more a confused, almost punitive act than an effort animated by the hope of discovery.

I am referring to the anger we feel as teachers working with students limited and constrained by our failure, as the generation who came before, to provide history and context to their present lives, a language of possibility, or a vision of hope for their future day.

I am referring to the anger we feel as citizens in a society described by the poet Maya Angelou as "bloody days and frightful nights when an urban warrior can find no face more despicable than his own, no ammunition more deadly than self-hate and no target more deserving of his true aim than his brother."

I am referring to the anger we feel as women "in this terrifying and murderous season, when young women achieve adulthood before puberty, and become mothers before learning how to be daughters" (Angelou).

I am referring to the anger we feel as citizens reading in the newspapers each morning of an unemployment rate that rises continuously—reading figures that project that an average of 5,600 Americans will lose their jobs each day in 1992.

Finally, I am referring to the anger we feel when we come to realize that "The tragedy of modern man," in the words of Vaclav Havel, "is not that he knows less and less about the meaning of his own life, but that it bothers him less and less." (1989, p. 237.)

While a program on the issues and opportunities for gerontological nursing in the twenty-first century might not, on first consideration, seem a logical place to discuss such anger, I argue that only as we come together to talk about our anger will we be enabled or, in the current parlance, *empowered* to advance our visions of a more humane society.

ABOUT POWER

On the other hand, discussion of power might seem even less appropriate for a program about those needing long-term care—those who, on first thought, are not among the powerful. In this regard, I will take this opportunity to discuss a kind of power that differs from the traditional discussion of power.

The power I ask you to consider is not the power of definition and exclusion wielded by the patriarchy to reinforce its position of dominance and authority by positioning itself and its values as the central point against which all others are measured.

Nor is it the constricting power of traditional science which, by definition, limits itself to empirical knowledge. We are warned against such limited knowledge and such restrictive science by the Union of Italian

Women, contemporary feminists who, in reaction to the Chernobyl incident, reminded us that "Power will pay dearly for its arrogance / Science will pay dearly for its ignorance" (1991, p. 337).

Nor is it the destructive power of violence, the negative force that builds and threatens our civilization—and upon which our health care system is also built. There is little health for us in a health care system that is built on the violent commandment of "Find the microbe and kill it" (Shaw).

Nor do I refer to the power of silence that pervades the research community as the powers that be bury their heads in the sand while the growing epidemic of HIV infections threatens the lives of ever increasing numbers of women, men, infants, and children.

Nor do I refer to the power of division that obfuscates the real and determining relationships that exist between poverty and disease, between a depressed economy and increasingly pathological communities, or between political philosophies and a creeping national ennui.

Nor do I suggest that we spend any time at all talking about the power of individuals—this is not a paper on heroes or heroines.

Rather, there is the power that flows from feminism, a power integral to a very specific consciousness of the oppression of women and a very special resistance to their oppression.

There is the inclusive and ever expanding feminist definition of power as presented by Chinn and Wheeler in their classic *Peace and Power,* the power of process, of letting go, of the whole, of collectivity, of unity, of sharing, of integration, of nurturing, of distribution, of intuition, of consciousness, of diversity, and of responsibility.

I ask you to attend to the idea of power as described by Bevis as "power to," or to the energizing power of women sharing the stories of their lives that Le Sueur describes as "Power without the use of wires."

This is the same power that the contemporary writer Carolyn Heilburn talks about in her recent work *Writing a Woman's Life:* "Power is the ability to take one's place in whatever discourse is essential to action and the right to have one's part matter" (1988, p. 18).

The power I ask us to ponder is the power of friendship—not a romantic and nostalgic friendship—but a friendship such as existed among the architects of the Cold War, who "Secure in their common outlook, empowered by the bonds of trust, . . . met the challenge of a demanding new age. In their sense of duty and shared wisdom they found the force to shape the world" (Issacson & Thomas, 1986, p. 741).

Such power is that of male friendship transformed by women who "share the wonderful energy of work in the public sphere" (Heilburn,

p. 108). It is the power inherent in the friendship among women, described by Janice Raymond in *A Passion for Friends*, as ". . . an ongoing testament and testimony of women as acting subjects who, in relation to their vital Selves and each other, have created passion, purpose and politics" (p. 21).

It is the power of our differences and our diversity celebrated and exalted.

NURSING'S AGENDA FOR HEALTH CARE REFORM

In writing about anger and power, Audre Lorde says: "anger expressed and translated into action in the service of our vision and our future is a liberating and strengthening act of clarification . . ." (1984, p. 127).

What is our vision, the vision to be served by our anger and our power? What is the vision of feminist nurses? I suggest to you that nursing's vision has been clarified most distinctly, probably more distinctly than at any time in our history, by the agenda for health care reform that is currently being proposed by organized nursing.

For perhaps the first time in nursing's history, we have presented the country with a clear vision of how to actualize our dreams that we are a nation committed to the health of all its people. By introducing a national campaign to advance "Nursing's Agenda for Health Care Reform" into the public arena, nursing both delineates itself from the current system and sets the stage for a decisive moment in the history of health care.

Nursing's agenda for health care reform calls for a radical restructuring of the health care system to such an extent that it will be as different from what we know now as apples are from bananas:

- *Primary care* rather than acute care will be the hub of the wheel.
- Primary care will be *delivered closer* to where the individuals live and work—in schools, at worksites, in nursing centers, and in long-term care facilities rather than where providers house their technology.
- A range of *alternative providers* who have been educated to collaborate with patients and their families in making decisions about their health care will be available.

- All providers will be *reimbursed directly* for their services.
- Financing will come from a *mix* of contributions from government, employers, insurance, and individuals with mechanisms in place to protect against excessive and catastrophic costs.
- Most important for our reforms is the value central to all others—the consumers are in charge; the consumers, rather than the professionals, *own* their own care; the consumers *own* their own health; and the consumers, rather than the physicians, and even nurses, *own* their own experiences.

RESEARCH NEEDED FOR NURSING'S AGENDA

While some still hold to the notion that science is a neutral enterprise, there is growing recognition that science, as a distinct ideology, reflects the values and mores of a culture. Any science—and the research conducted in the name of science—functions to legitimate both itself and something more. Science is one of the central means and conduits of the hegemonic creep by which a culture's values infiltrate into all spheres of life—in both public and private spheres.

As expected, the science of our culture reflects the values, the dualities, and the polarities too generously defined by men. It is a science of dominance and control, of prediction and precision, a science that builds and supports the technology capable of "precision" bombing of smokestacks and "surgical" air strikes. It is a science that is also limited in its understanding of the effect of its technologies of war on the lives and the deaths of Iraqi women and children and Kurdish families.

The prevailing science—and the research conducted in its name—can create and extend life, can transplant organs, and can split genetic materials. But such a science is painfully limited when we send those little babies home, for example, when we turn to understand the life lived via machines, or when we read of the African men who sell their kidneys to international traders so that their families can eat.

A reformed health care system will have little use for this information of power and control since it calls for a radical restructuring of the power relationships that currently exist.

The power of process, of collectivity, and of friendship that I spoke of before is the power needed for a reformed health care system. In

Heilburn's words such "power consists to a large extent in deciding what stories will be told; . . . as male power has made certain stories unthinkable" (1988, p. 44).

The power that is needed for the new health care system will be found in the stories not yet told. There is great power embedded in the knowledge of discovery of women's values and the uncovering of women's lives. It is the knowledge that Virginia Satir talked about when she urged us to make the covert overt, the hidden obvious, and the implicit explicit.

Such stories to be uncovered tell of how to care and nurture the life forces within us. They speak of a knowledge that is not of one truth or one reality, but a knowledge that roots in the diversity of our lives. These are the stories of our differences, the stories of what it means to be of color in a white world, from the East in a world dominated by the values of Western Europe, or from the South in a world dominated by the North.

These are the stories of what it means to be poor in the land of plenty, aging in the culture of youth, without meaningful work among the puritans, in a wheelchair in a world of narrow aisles and steps, or gay or lesbian among heterosexuals.

The knowledge needed is the knowledge of our choices as women and that women value, our choice to have or not to have children, to love or not love men, to love or not love women.

From here is where the power to change the world will come.

From here is where the inspiration for our visions will come. From these stories, from this frame of reference, from this multidimensional understanding of our relationship to the aging in our society will come the substance of our visions.

Here, therefore, is where we should situate our scholarship and research—in the stories of our aging, the stories of those working in long-term facilities, the stories of those living in long-term care facilities.

Le Sueur provides us with the inspiration to tell these stories, to be witness:

> *Perhaps women like me of another generation are a bridge. Pass over, use the energy of the root in our witness and our singing. So we will never be gone. You have more tools now. The fog is lifting over the illusions. You have begun to tell it. You will bear sharper witness. Be bold. Tell it all. Don't spare the horses. The earth is waiting to hear you. All the children and the ancients are waiting. We shall come home together* (1982, p. 291).

ABOUT RISKS

Before closing, I would like to say a few words about risks, about the risks involved in all this anger, all this power, about the risks involved in presenting such a clear vision and such clarification.

The wisdom of the *I Ching* tells us that "The price of increasing power is increasing opposition."

There is, of course, a very common reaction to be expected when women express their anger. Heilburn tells how women writing about anger are dismissed as "shrill and strident women." Virginia Woolf warns of ". . . the ridicule, misery and anxiety the patriarchy holds in store for those who express their anger about the enforced destiny of women." And Audre Lorde forewarns us that we will be "accused of destruction."

There is an inherent excitement in the realization that the realities created through the conversations of feminists and nurses will differ radically from the realities that are presented to us daily under the banner of "but that's just the way things are." These realities we create will differ profoundly from those presented by the advocating agents of science and technology; they will differ in the most fundamental ways from the realities created by those who still embrace, despite the fact that it is increasingly decrepit and dysfunctional, the biomedical paradigm within which the Western world has constructed its research agenda and its health care systems.

As you are undoubtedly aware, there is also an inherent risk in challenging the status quo by including feelings and subjectivity into the factual and objective world of science. In addition to the inherent risks of being seen as deviant, there is the risk to our egos of appearing as not scientific enough or intelligent enough to be considered a "real" researcher, the risk to our careers of having our work evaluated as too soft or too subjective to merit funding or publication. There is even the risk, if you accept some of the recent arguments in the literature, that nursing might not, in fact, be a science.

Thus, as you consider our discussions of anger and power and the risks inherent in both, we will as nurses create new ways of knowing our shared realities. While I haven't the clearest of notions of exactly what those ways will be or exactly what that knowledge will be, I am forever invigorated by the realization that, in the process, the realities we create will be our own realities:

- The realities of angry women who refuse to take the given as destiny.

- The realities of empowered women who "share the wonderful energy of work in the public sphere."
- The realities of nurses who have taken health and healing as our life projects.
- The realities within which peace will grow and absorb the need for anger.
- The realities within which peace will embrace the power of friendship.
- Not an absolute reality or an absolute truth.
- Not a single vision for long-term care.
- But the only reality, among the many realities.
- The only vision among the many visions.
- The only one that is worth the risk.

REFERENCES

Angelou, M. (1991, August 25). I dare to hope. *The New York Times*, Section 4, p. 15.

Bateson, G. (1972). *Steps to an ecology of mind.* New York: Ballantine Books.

Bevis, E. O., & Watson, J. (1989). *Toward a caring curriculum.* New York: National League for Nursing.

Center for Defense Information. (1991, May/June). The economy of death. Washington, DC: The Author, p. 15.

Fisher, M. F. K. (1984). *Sister age.* New York: Vintage Books.

Havel, V. (1989). *Letters to Olga.* P. Wilson (Trans.). New York: Henry Holt and Company.

Heilburn, C. (1988). *Writing a woman's life.* New York: Ballantine Books.

Issacson & Thomas. (1986). *The wise men. Six friends and the world they made.* New York: Simon and Schuster.

Klare, M. (1991, June 3). High-death weapons of the Gulf War. *The Nation*, pp. 738–742.

Le Suere, M. (1982). *Ripening.* New York: The Feminist Press of The City of New York.

Lorde, A. (1984). *Sister outsider.* Freedom, CA: The Crossing Press.

Raymond, J. G. (1986). *A passion for friends: Toward a philosophy of female affection.* Boston: Beacon Press.

Sarton, M. (1988). *After the stroke: A journal.* New York: W. W. Norton and Company.

Union of Italian Women, La Goccia, Rome. (1991). In Bono, Paola, & Kemp (Eds.), *Italian feminist thought: A reader.* Oxford: Basil Blackwell.

Wheeler, C., & Chinn, P. (1988). *Peace and power: A handbook of feminist process.* New York: National League for Nursing.

9

A Symphony of Caring: Shared Visions and Eloquent Futures for Nursing Education and Practice

Em Olivia Bevis

I. INTRODUCTION

The title "A Symphony of Caring: Shared Visions and Eloquent Futures for Nursing Education and Practice" sets a task for me to examine how, due to the caring imperative for nursing, nursing practice and education share the same vision of the future and are obliged to create an alliance for bringing that future about.

The title conjures images of music, harmony, insights, and accord. Music of the Classical and early Romantic Eras, written by Hayden, Mozart, Schubert, Beethoven, and Brahms, brings to mind the sonata form in which these composers wrote. The term "sonata-allegro form," often used to describe the first movement of classical symphonies and various forms of chamber music, is comprised of five distinct parts. Part one introduces and sets the stage for what is to follow. Part two is the exposition in which a primary theme is followed by a second theme in a different but related key and is concluded with a short section. Part three comprises the development in which one or more themes of the exposition are elaborated. Part four recapitulates, repeating the exposition but with some modifications. Last, part five is the coda, or the concluding portion, which is usually brief.

This chapter follows these same five components of the classical sonata-allegro form.

II. EXPOSITION OF A THEME FOLLOWED BY A SECOND THEME IN A DIFFERENT THOUGH RELATED KEY AND A SHORT CONCLUDING SECTION

The First Theme: Caring

The major theme, caring, is a demanding theme, with layers of meaning heard only when one listens carefully. The second theme, in a different but related key, is a vision of part of nursing's future—played in a minor key to denote the magic of expectations.

Caring is the essence of nursing. In her 1988 book *Nursing: Human Science and Human Care*, Watson speaks of caring as the moral ideal of nursing. A moral ideal is compelling. It is an overriding influence that demands commitment and reflective actions regarding things concerning the ideal. A moral ideal is the motor that runs the system. Noddings (1984) calls caring a "moral imperative." An imperative is a command, a will to influence behavior, an obligatory act that cannot be avoided or evaded. As nursing's ethical ideal and moral imperative, caring has certain distinctive qualities.

First, it obligates or compels one to act for, with, and on behalf of the one or ones cared about (Murray & Bevis, 1989). Second, this action is guided by a moral disposition to do good. Noddings (1984) describes this moral disposition as a longing after good that leads to a sense of ethics, which sense then guides the doing of good for those cared for. Gaut (1983), as one of the three conditions that are both necessary and sufficient for caring, speaks of a positive change occurring as a result of caring and adds that change is judged solely on the basis of the welfare of others. When using words such as *positive*, *welfare*, and *judging*, values immediately become apparent, which again confronts us with Noddings's moral longing after good—but good as judged by whom or what? The answer may lie in the goals of caring. Mayeroff (1971) describes caring as helping the ones cared about grow and actualize themselves. Similarly, Fromm (1956), in speaking of loving in a way that makes it seem very like caring, describes it as "active concern for the life and growth of that which we love" (p. 26). The key element here is clear: it is that which seeks to help those cared about grow toward self-actualization and, further, to the realization of their greatest potential. It is this drive to improve the human condition, to enable the maximizing of the good, that will ultimately force nurses to assume the general reshaping of the role of caring in society as well as the reshaping of the greater health care system itself.

The nature of that goodness, that moral and ethical action that caring engenders, is noteworthy. There are several elements that characterize its expression. Examining caring writers and theorists such as Fromm (1956), Gaut (1979), Leininger (1978), Mayeroff (1971), Murray and Bevis (1989), Noddings (1984), Ray (1978), and Watson (1988), there also emerge common characteristics that have congruence. Each of these characteristics describes the kind of care required, not only by our elderly, but by all of the population; the elderly, of course, are among the most needy and neglected by nursing and other health care providers.

Probably the most pervasive theme here is that caring is an active force that compels or obligates one to powerfully positive acts based on thoughts and feelings of love, affection, and deep commitment to the one cared for. While some of these themes have been described with rare beauty in preceding chapters, other themes that support this central thesis are:

1. Presence and availability.
2. Receptivity/attendance.
3. Trust/honesty.
4. Responsibility.
5. Personalization as opposed to objectification.
6. Touch/affection.
7. Empathy/being in cared one's personal framework.
8. Helping/sharing of motive energy/nurturance and succorance.
9. Assisting in human need gratification.
10. Intimacy, expression of feelings, involvement, and providing time and space for seeing and feeling.
11. Respect.

These common elements provide us a feel for and insights into the possible structure of caring as a universal human phenomenon of central importance to nursing. Notice that all of the characteristics listed have to do with individual-to-individual caring. There is little emphasis on cure-related environments and their ethic, power relationships, political and economic conditions, and the feminine oppression that is part of the societal hegemony that inhibits nurse caring. (This theme will be amplified in part three, the development.)

Second Theme in a Different but Related Key: Shared Visions and Eloquent Futures

Sharing a vision and building an eloquent future based on that vision requires that practice and education become allied so as to make sharing possible. Such alliances can grow from a common cause, for the whole of nursing, practice and education, moves in the ways and in the directions that visionaries and theorists lead. There are melodious motifs in the visions that abound in the literature. These visions revolve around paradigm shifts for practice and education, with nurses focusing on *nursing* work, providing patient-clients with wide options and choices, making caring work valued and legitimate, respecting the wholeness and integrity of humans, graduating the professional level nurse, and bringing care, not just cure, to society.

The Vision of the Paradigm Shift. Newman, Sime, and Corcoran-Perry (1991), in examining the focus of the discipline of nursing, maintain that, "a discipline is distinguished by a domain of inquiry that represents a shared belief among its members regarding its reason for being" (p. 1). Bypassing other distinguishing indicators of a discipline to concentrate on this and citing extensive research, conferences, and nursing literature of the last ten years, they propose that nursing's specific domain or focus is the study of caring in the health experience. They also suggest that nurse caring is transforming, and like other caring theorists and researchers they connect caring, healing, and health (Watson, 1979, 1985, 1990; Leininger, 1984; Benner, 1988). This requires that we refocus our energy toward our true domain, caring during the health care experience.

The Vision of Nurses Focusing on Nursing Work. Turning the perspective on the subject half a turn, we have a reconceptualization of the work place occurring via demographics and altered views of the focus of nursing. This reconceptualization confronts us with the cure-care dichotomy of nursing practice. Not only is the world population aging, which alone is a major influencing factor on nursing, but nurses, as mentioned above, are realizing that their true focus is on care, not cure (Gadow, 1988; Watson, 1990; Newman et al., 1991), and that acute hospitals concentrate on technology or what Watson (1979) calls the "trim" of nursing. This "trim," or technological focus, is especially valued in acute-care institutions beyond its real or essential value and as such receives all work place rewards associated with nursing success. As we know, the work place as currently lived places little value and few rewards on caring, as compared with curing. Tagliareni et al. (1991) address this issue while speaking of nursing homes. They say: "Because the nursing home setting is less focused on cure oriented technology and more focused on maintenance and rehabilitative interventions, nursing practice is less structured. The technically focused, acute-care practitioner is no longer the expert" (p. 3). Because it is so obvious in the nursing home setting, they help us to see that our tradition of cure-focused acute-care emphasis in nursing education is limiting and outmoded. But let us be specific here. It is not that nursing care is not required in cure; it is, but the role of nursing in cure is secondary and self-limiting. Care, not cure, within the health experience is the distinguishing characteristic and the moral imperative of nursing (Watson, 1988; Gadow, 1988; Newman et al., 1991).

The Vision of Making Caring Work Valued and Legitimate. Unfortunately, nurses have taken on the physician's position that cure is the highest calling. In this regard, Gadow (1988), Watson (1988), and Bevis (1991) maintain that caring involves an ethic as high or even higher than curing. Gadow (1988), for one, proposes that "care is an end in itself. While it may serve as a means of reaching a further state, it is always and above all a state that itself can be fully inhabited. While it may serve as a vessel for reaching a remote shore, it is at the same time and above all a vessel in which one can live even when—especially when—there is no destination in sight or in mind" (pp. 5–6). What we must realize, however, is that medicine has the professional goal of curing and that nursing adopted that goal. Nursing also adopted the idea that, failing to cure, the role of nurses was to assist the individual to "a peaceful death." This places little value on nursing that is neither for cure nor for easy death.

Care of the elderly and being the care giver in nursing homes, however, offer the unique and special privilege to nurses of practicing their highest state: caring, with no other destination or end in sight. Settings placing less value on caring may, in the future, be compelled to emulate such quality of care by placing more emphasis on the specific role of caring to entice nurses to participate more in curing—or put another way—on the technical aspects.

Watson (1988), in addressing nursing's method, speaks of transcendental phenomenology. She says, "if phenomenology is to be true to the human science and art of nursing and the human care process, it must penetrate beneath the surface of the familiar, habitually organized, and standardized experience . . . . The process of transcendental phenomenology commits us to a language that encourages existential authenticity" (p. 91). Here, in one stroke of the pen, she did away with "nursing process," "nursing diagnosis," and a multitude of misguided governmental attempts at regulation and cost control that rest on standardized categories of objectified persons, such as diagnostic related groupings and patient classification systems. This certainly reconceptualizes practice and points up the re-personalization of nursing that Tagliareni addressed in her chapter.

MacPherson (1991) visualizes a utopian world where caring has been socialized.

> *Caring at all levels—be it child care, illness care or elderly care is viewed as a societal responsibility. Caring in this envisioned future becomes the highest ethical concern of being human. Women and men inclined to practice caring professionally choose to be care workers with good pay and high status. Gender and class problems fade away to allow nurses to have the kind of caring relationship with clients described by Leininger (1984), Watson, (1979, 1987, 1988), Noddings (1984), Roberts (1990), and others. Such a professional goal attains broad societal support (p. 37).*

MacPherson proposes that "socialization of caring work, particularly with our aging population, is an utopian idea whose time has come."

Both Roberts (1990) and Watson (1990) propose that nursing's core value, caring, must be translated into public policy. Public policy, then, must be used to reconceputalize the work place so that the vision of making nursing work valued and legitimate can be realized.

Other visions are shared: nurses practicing with autonomy, nurses learning to think critically, nurses influencing health policy, and nurses practicing in ways that acknowledge the lived reality of patients' wholeness, their need for inner and outer harmony, and their need for transforming caring relationships—where the meaning of care in the human health experience is played out on the stage of reality.

Short Concluding Section

Caring in the human health experience is the compelling mission of nursing. This mission is thwarted by nurses' own lack of clarity regarding their domain of practice and by the economic and power issues within the context and systems in which they work. This compelling mission necessitates nurses creating a shared vision of nursing's future so that such a vision can become reality. In the words of Oscar Hammerstein II (*South Pacific*), "if you never have a dream, you never have a dream come true."

III. DEVELOPMENT—WHEREIN ONE OR MORE THEMES OF THE EXPOSITION ARE DEVELOPED

The two themes of the exposition, nursing's caring focus and shared visions and futures, require that we examine some of the factors that inhibit our ability to enact our caring mandate and build the future we envision. Here we follow the natural flow of the music.

Development 1: Factors Affecting Nurses' Ability To Care

Examining nursing's shared belief and focus statement that "nursing is the study of caring in the human health experience" (Newman et al., p. 3) provokes a shared vision, a vision yet inhibited by the hegemony of privilege and power. It follows that social transformation of the health system context for caring, the nurse's ability to provide caring in that milieu, and the alteration of the power relationships in that context become the tasks of nurses who care. To do this caring for the vulnerable, child care, illness care, elderly care, and preventive care becomes a social responsibility with (as Moccia has pointed out in her chapter) power relationships as the major issue that must be dealt with in order for caring to be provided. Some of these economic, power, and gender issues that curb our ability to implement our caring mandate are examined here.

Bureaucracy and Profit. According to Salmon (1987), the number of independent health care agencies is diminishing and megacorporations are spiraling as large investor-owned for-profit corporations have taken over many acute-care hospitals, nursing homes, and health maintenance organizations. Nurses and other health care workers, working in settings in these profit-generating megacorporations, have had their care negatively influenced by the emphasis on profit and the depersonalization common to large bureaucracies. Additionally, governmental attempts to control costs have hit nursing hard—sometimes as an unanticipated outcome of policies that nurses were not allowed to help shape. According to MacPherson (1991), the nonphysician workers in the health care system are divided into over 375 independent occupations. She adds that most of these are low-wage, dead-end positions. "This process of continually bifurcating labor so as to parcel it out to a single worker is a general tendency of modern capitalism" (p. 35). Citing Braverman (1974), MacPherson maintains that this fragmentation is not done to increase efficiency but to maximize management control over labor and to replace highly skilled costly workers with less skilled, cheaper labor. All of this is detrimental to patients and to the health of the nation.

Power, Gender, and Economics in Caring. Another factor influencing our ability to care is power, which is intertwined with gender and economics. In the light of the politics of caring that skews power relationships so that job fragmentation and reduction of skill are not only allowed but rewarded through government and public policy, one can see that nurse "shortages" probably exist, as Macpherson (1991) says, not so much from the opening of other professions, but because of the organization, administration, and structure of care found in the U.S. health care system. She states, "As we are recognizing, along with the public, that caring is a central ethic of nursing, we are also recognizing that our ability to operationalize this ethic is being seriously undermined by the social context in which we practice" (p. 25). She states further, "the current paradigm stresses individual motivation for caring while ignoring both the material conditions and the power relations in the contexts where nurses work" (p. 27).

Another constraining element is the economics of caring. As seen by Noddings (1984) and Ward (1991), caring is feminine. Noddings (1984) refers to caring as feminine in the deep classical sense—rooted in receptivity, relatedness, and responsiveness. It is not that men do not or should not embrace caring; it is that caring belongs to the feminine nature of things and is seen by society as women's work. As women's work, it is also underpaid and undervalued (Riverby, 1987).

Ward (1991), in describing "kin care," which she defines as care of the frail elderly at home by largely female relatives, maintains that it is not considered work because it is not seen as work. It is not seen as work because it is underpaid and done by women. Since it is not classified as work, it is not figured into health care cost nor is it computed into the gross national product. Ward (1991) computed the value of caregiving hours based on a 1982 national survey of caregivers to the frail elderly (Stone et al., 1986). Seventy-two percent of the survey responders were women providing an average of four hours per day of care and, according to Ward (1991), doing this in addition to a full-time job. Three-fourths of the sample provided care seven days a week. Extrapolating this to a population of approximately 2.2 million caregivers amounts to about 2,712,160,000 hours of care at the hourly wage of a home health aide—which is approximately $4.00 per hour—the work-worth of the care is $10,848,640,000.

If such care had been given by a home health aide agency, reimbursement costs would equal $17,629,040,000. Ward (1991) provides the information that "the replacement cost for a year of unpaid caregiving—is greater than the 1982 federal budget for Medicare payments for medical (not hospital) services . . . [or] almost half the budget-breaking federal Medicare payment in 1982 to hospitals." This represents a worst-case scenario of underpayment and undervaluing caring. And it points up the economics and invisibility of female caregiving labor.

There is another economic and gender-related issue to be considered when examining the oppression of caregivers and the suppression of caring. According to Waters (1991), 75 percent of nursing home residents are female. When one considers that these largely female residents are cared for by a largely female population of caregivers—many with one year or less of training—then we cannot ignore the fact that the care of the aged is a woman's issue. Being women and for the most part powerless, both the nursing home residents and the care providers are left to deal with the results of medicine's ability to prolong life without preserving life quality. It is the nurses, mostly female, in the nursing home setting and the mostly female caregivers at home who are concerned with life quality, or helping patients with their lived experiences with health. One can speculate that perhaps the fact that nursing homes are places where mostly women give care to mostly women has something to do with the fact that society at large (read medical, industrial, and political power-privilege persons) have substituted regulation (it is one of the most regulated of industries) for support of the real issues, the caring issues, that affect the lives of both residents and caregivers.

We are reminded by Nolin (1991) that "residents do not go to nursing homes to die, they go to live out their lives." This compels us, practitioners and educators alike, to provide care that, as Gadow (1988) says, has no other destination or end in sight. Caring for the frail elderly challenges us to hallow life, living, reality, and care and to exercise the power to reshape social and health policy to make this possible.

Development 2: A Coalition of Caring

A realliance among the factions of nursing that are generally given to horizontal violence is required if nursing is to fulfill its caring mission. Two of these adversarial groups are mentioned here.

First, education itself must heal its breaches and form a new alliance so that together we can build a different future. This means associate degree nursing and baccalaureate degree nursing—in fact, all forms of generic education—must beat their swords into plowshares. There is no room for the horizontal violence that has plagued the educational ranks. As Waters has reminded us on several occasions, diversity is healthy for the profession and, as identified in this book, collaboration works.

Next, practice and education must unite. Factionalism in nursing has and does absorb our energy and diverts us from our societal mission. Educators have spent time and energy on esoteric, personal prejudices, such as entry into practice, instead of the world-threatening problems of the health of the people in an exploited and damaged environment. Nursing practice and nursing education have argued and blamed each other over the trivia of who is responsible for the graduate's ability to practice upon graduation, rather than getting on with the task of seeing that they can practice. Membership on a few committees, attending a few meetings with each other, and sharing a few joint appointments does not accomplish an alliance. Caring demands a joint effort to change society. To do this, we must become united and allied—allies with the permission to be involved in one another's affairs as do friends who have the common value of caring about society. I am happy that collaboration is now occurring in new and wonderful ways—collaboration in nursing education, collaboration in forming a more hospitable work place, collaboration in transforming the sick-care system we have in the United States to a real health care system, and collaboration for and on behalf of our patients, our students, and ourselves.

This takes us into the final thrust of this symphony, praxis, critical thinking, and doing caring for society.

IV: RECAPITULATION: A REPEAT OF THE EXPOSITION WITH SOME MODIFICATION

Making the Shared Vision into an Eloquent Future

At the beginning of this chapter, proposed themes were caring and a shared vision of nursing's future. The recapitulation suggests that the shared vision can be made real through nurses working in caring concert to alter the assumptions, framework, and traditions of the health care system. This requires a change in both generic and staff development educational practices, for in order for caring nurses to change the world they must become critically conscious of the society in which they live, aware of the insidious nature of the hegemony of the powerful medical-industrial complex, and plan and execute counterhegemony toward the end of nursing's shared vision.

Transformative Empowerment. There is a connection between caring and the new nursing trends that emerges through the empowerment element. Caring, according to Murray and Bevis (1989), compels one to action for and on behalf of the one cared about. That caring has as end-in-view the emergence of the highest self possible, the realization of potential for the one cared for. That being true, caring is a natural progression to the realization that that highest self must be a self free of coercion and oppression, a self of personal and collective power.

Riverby (1987) and MacPherson (1991) make observations that are similar when examining caring through feminist perspectives. MacPherson states that acknowledging that the nurse's right to care should be equal to the physician's right to cure, though valid, fails to consider that "the individualism and autonomy promised by this rights framework often fails to acknowledge collective social need, to provide a way for adjudicating conflicts over rights, or to address the reasons for the devaluing of female activity" (p. 30). Riverby, saying much the same, also observes that "nurses have often rejected liberal feminism, not out of their oppression or some kind of 'false consciousness,' but because of some deep understandings of the limited promise of equality and autonomy in a health care system they see as flawed and harmful" (p. 207).

If that promise has failed, it makes it doubly important that we do not. This leaves nursing with the task of righting social wrongs or, to paraphrase Greene (1990), of creating some order in a disrupted health experience (p. 34). Greene affirms "caring as the ground of ethical existence" (p. 29) and uses this affirmation to observe that one is discussing care "in a fearfully care*less* society. Administered, systematized, bureaucratized, violent as it is, such society requires of us a deliberate resistance to many of its dominant values" (p. 29). Perhaps, resistance is too passive a word—a better effort would be that we deliberately plan to transform the traditions and values within which American society operates, and in so doing, transform society. Enraged as we are by the lack of caring in the health care system, our own caring as the ground of our ethical existence compels us to act in ways that alter society. For this obligation I am suggesting two things: (1) that nurses be taught the art of praxis and (2) that as a component of praxis, nurses be taught critical thinking through a critical theory and a feminist viewpoint in order to know how to exercise power to alter the traditions of health care system practices.

Praxis. The concept of praxis ties in with all the pivotal factors necessary for nurses to achieve a societal vision.

First, it is connected with transforming society. Praxis does this by transforming the assumptions and the framework of traditions and expectations within which the field operates (Carr & Kemmis, 1986) (e.g., the reconstruction of the fundamental character of the social setting of nursing and health care). Second, praxis is guided by the moral disposition to act truly, justly, and caringly. This ties in with Murray and Bevis's (1989) compelling or obligatory action aspect of caring and is rooted in Noddings's (1984) longing after good.

Carr and Kemmis (1986) explain it this way: "Craft or technical knowledge is not reflexive; it does not change the framework of tradition and expectation within which it operates. Nor does it take the view that, through the exercise of the craft, the fundamental character of the social setting will be reconstructed. *Praxis,* however, does have this character—it remakes the conditions of informed action and constantly reviews action and the knowledge which informs it" (p. 33). Praxis is reflective action.

Critical Thinking. Praxis requires critical thinking, and critical thinking—poorly understood and seldom taught—is rooted in critical consciousness. Critical consciousness is awareness of the world assessed against some criteria based on values, values that have social worth at the core and a better world as the goal. These values include emancipation, concern, compassion and caring, quality of life (for all), the best possible use of resources, and egalitarianism (equality of participation, responsibility, and benefits). Critical consciousness also requires an awareness of the subtle ways awareness itself is obscured and our criticality is inhibited. It is a practiced skill that with use gradually drops the veils from our eyes and allows us to see the way factors within the social organization, such as morays and folkways, mask and prevent the valued ideals from occurring. Critical consciousness enables one to see the assumptions on which normative ways of being are premised and the assumptions that underlie the assumptions, so that not only are the philosophical structures on which social phenomena are based more obvious, but so too are the consequences.

It is the nature of praxis that it can best be practiced by people who think critically. Critical thinking, however, can be better described than defined. People who think critically have certain characteristics in common.

First and foremost is critical consciousness that makes one sensitive to the hegemonically constructed world of health care. Hegemony is the way individuals and institutions saturate society and individual consciousness with beliefs that maintain the status quo of power and privilege. Hegemonically constructed perceptions constitute what is "common sense" to most people. It becomes our perceived "only world." Apple (1979) describes it as "an organized assemblage of meaning and practices—the central, effective, and dominant system of meanings, values, and actions which are lived."

Bevis (1991b) proposes that "Educational institutions and educators act as part of this process of saturation, for hegemony dictates what we learn as history, what we see as significant, what we are conscious of, and how we view our place in society and our expectations. The realty we admit into consciousness is confirming of that hegemonistically constituted reality, for we put evidence through a screen conditioned by socially structured hegemony" (pp. 4–5).

As an aside, I would like to point out that the underutilization and misuse of nursing homes in nursing education is due in large part to hegemonically constructed values. We choose acute medical centers, acute illness, medical diagnosis, and nursing's dependent roles as being the "truths" that best fit the needs of our students and graduates for serving in the current hegemonically influenced "reality." We seem unable to shake loose the conditioned knowledge of what is real, practical, common sense, and effective and attain a different awareness of reality.

Returning to critical thinking, critical consciousness, and hegemony, Bevis (1992) describes critical thinkers as listed below and states that such thinkers are critically conscious and have strategies for countering hegemony. They are aware of and emancipated from personal, institutional, environmental, political, and social *hegemony* that programs thinking. To do this they:

- Are aware of media bias, distortion, and influence.
- Are free of dogma.
- Admit to and respect the possibilities and validity of multiple belief systems.
- Are open to alternative ways of viewing and being in the world.
- Make their own judgments and decisions—not allowing others to do it for them.

Further, critical thinkers:

- Are aware of *assumptions* under which we and others think and act.
- Have insight into the *assumptions* under those *assumptions*.
- Are motivated and driven by an ethical and moral longing after good.
- Encourage diversity.
- Take responsibility for their own actions and for their ability to influence the course of events.
- Acknowledge change as a fundamental reality.
- Confront existing *reality* and dream of and construct other realities.
- Are reflective, action oriented, socially transforming, and compelled to caring, compassionate deeds (practice praxis).
- Are committed to and have a sense of community connectedness.
- See *patterns*.
- Recognize *significance*.
- Seek *meanings* (even after some have been found).
- In solving problems critical thinkers are:
  - *wary* of absolutes
  - *viewers* of wholes in their context
  - *skeptical* of formulistic answers and responses
  - *suspicious* of quick-fix solutions
  - *leery* of universal truths

- *distrustful* of single cause-effect or simplistic answers
- *creative* in generating options, alternatives, and strategies
- *seekers* of win/win solutions
- *anticipatory*: can project where a course of action and lines of thinking lead and therefore anticipate rather than face crisis
- *avoiders* of stasis
- In human relationships (personal and professional) critical thinkers:
  - *empower* others—believe in "power to" rather than "power over"
  - *establish* egalitarian partnerships with others
  - *have* a sense of community and common destiny with all humankind
  - *enter* into dialectical rather than polemic discussions
  - *are* more interested in exploring possible "truths" than in defending a posited "truth"

V. CODA—THE CONCLUDING PORTION

For the coda, literally the "tail," I have chosen to quote Maxine Greene who spoke at the 11th International Caring Conference in Denver in 1989. "When I speak of the 'passions' of caring, paradoxical though it may seem . . . I have wide-awakeness in mind; I have in mind a going up against the abstract, the domesticating, the systematized. Only then are there likely to be the collaborative actions intended to transform."

She goes on to say: "I believe that caring must be deliberately achieved, as freedom must be achieved. It is going to take thoughtfulness, courage, and desire to do so—an opening of spaces where we can truly care. It is going to take political action now and then within and outside our institutions. And it may take poetry and serendipitous visions, and music, and even painting for the sake of empowering persons to hear and see what is often behind the veil."

This, then, is the prescription for our task. We cannot allow the existential realities of persons in health experiences to be defined by medical diagnosis, to be confined by parameters of role or nursing diagnosis, or to be distorted by marginal existence in poverty, gender, age, or fragile vulnerability. This is the role of a civilized people: to care for its citizens. This is the social mandate for nurses.

BIBLIOGRAPHY

Benner, P. (1984). *From novice to expert: excellence and power in clinical nursing practice.* Menlo Park, CA: Addison-Wesley Publishing Co.

Benner, P. (1988). *Nursing as a caring profession.* Presented at the meeting of the American Academy of Nursing, October 16, 1988, Kansas City, MO.

Berrey, E. R. (1991). Researching the lives of eminent women in nursing: Rozella M. Schlotfeldt. In R.M. Neil and R. Watts (Eds.), *Caring and nursing: Explorations in feminist perspectives.* New York: National League for Nursing.

Bevis, E. O., & Watson, J. (1989) *Toward a caring curriculum: A new pedagogy for nursing.* New York: National League for Nursing.

Bevis, E. O. (1991a). The future for nursing education and nursing practice: An alliance for destiny. *Nursing Management.* In press.

Bevis, E. O. (1991b) *Escaping the Lotus Isles.* Unpublished.

Bevis, E. O. (1992). *Critical thinking.* Unpublished manuscript.

Carr, W., & Kemmis, S. (1986). *Becoming critical: Knowing through action research.* Geelong, Australia: Deakin University Press.

Fromm, E. (1956). *The art of loving: An enquiry into the nature of love.* New York: Harper and Brothers.

Gadow, S. (1988). Covenant without cure: Letting go and holding on in chronic illness. In J. Watson and M.A. Ray (Eds.), *The ethics of care and the ethics of cure: Synthesis in chronicicity.* New York: National League for Nursing.

Gaut, D. (1979). Conceptual analysis of caring: Research method. In M. Leininger (Ed.), (1981). *Caring, an essential human need: Proceedings of the three national caring conferences.* Thorofare, NJ: Slack.

Gaut, D. (1983). Development of a theoretically adequate description of caring. *Western Journal of Nursing Research.* 5(4), 313–324.

Greene, M. (1990). The tensions and passions of caring. In M. Leininger & J. Watson (Eds.), *The caring imperative in education.* New York: National League for Nursing.

Leininger, M. (1978). The phenomenon of caring: Importance, research questions and theoretical considerations. In M. Leininger (Ed.), *Caring, an essential human need: Proceedings of the three national caring conferences.* Thorofare, NJ: Slack.

Leininger, M. (1984). *Care: The essence of nursing and health.* Thorofare, NJ: Slack.

MacPherson, K. I. (1991). Looking at caring and nursing through a feminist lens. In R.M. Neil & R. Watts (Eds.), *Caring and nursing: Explorations in feminist perspectives.* New York: National League for Nursing.

Mayeroff, M. (1971). *On caring.* New York: Perennial Library.
Murray, J., & Bevis, E. (1989). In Bevis, E., *Curriculum building in nursing: A process.* New York: National League for Nursing.

Watson, J. (1990). The moral failure of the patriarchy. *Nursing Outlook, 38*(2), 62–67.

Mayeroff, M. (1971). *On caring.* New York: Perennial Library.
Murray, J., & Bevis, E. (1989). In Bevis, E., *Curriculum building in nursing: A process.* New York: National League for Nursing.
Newman, M.A., Sime, A.M, & Corcoran-Perry, S.A. (1991). The focus of the discipline of nursing. *Advances in Nursing Science, 14*(1), 1–6.
Noddings, N. (1984). *Caring: A feminine approach to ethics and moral education.* Berkley: University of California Press.
Nolin, J. (1991). *Letter to Aunt Em.* Unpublished.
Ray, M. (1978). A philosophical analysis of caring within nursing. In M. Leininger (Ed.), *Caring, an essential human need: Proceedings of the three national caring conferences.* Thorofare, NJ: Slack.
Riverby, S. (1987). *Ordered to care, the dilemma of American nursing, 1850–1945.* New York: Cambridge University Press.
Salmon, J. (1987). The medical profession and the corporatization of the health sector. *Theoretical Medicine, 8,* 19–29.
Stone, R., et al. (1986). *Caregivers of the frail elderly: A national profile.* Rockville, MD: Division of Intramural Research, National Center for Health Services Research and Health Care Technology Assessment.
Tagliareni, E., Sherman, S., Waters, V., & Mengel, A. (1991). Participatory clinical education: Reconceptualizing the clinical learning environment. *Nursing and Health Care.*
Ward, D. (1991). Gender and cost in caring. In R.M. Neil & R. Watts (Eds.), *Caring and nursing: Explorations in feminist perspectives.* New York: National League for Nursing.
Waters, V. (Ed.). (1991). *Teaching gerontology.* New York: National League for Nursing.
Watson, J. (1979). *Nursing: The philosophy and science of caring.* Boston: Little, Brown and Company.
Watson, J. (1987). Advancing the art and science of human caring. In *Proceedings of the Western Society of Research in Nursing conference, 20.* Boulder, CO: Western Institute of Nursing.
Watson, J. (1988). *Nursing: human science and human care: A theory of nursing.* New York: National League for Nursing.
Watson, J. (1990). The moral failure of the patriarchy. *Nursing Outlook, 38*(2), 62–67.